SURGERY FOR PHONATORY DISORDERS

Monographs In
Clinical Otolaryngology

VOLUME 3

SURGERY FOR PHONATORY DISORDERS

Harvey M. Tucker, M.D., F.A.C.S.
Chairman
Department of Otolaryngology
  and Communicative Disorders
Cleveland Clinic Foundation
Cleveland, Ohio

Illustrated by
James T. Suchy, A.M.I.

Churchill Livingstone
New York, Edinburgh, London, and Melbourne 1981

Distributed in the United Kingdom by Churchill Livingstone, Robert Stevenson House, 1-3 Baxter's Place, Leith Walk, Edinburgh EH1 3AF and by associated companies, branches and representatives throughout the world.

First published 1981
Printed in U.S.A.

ISBN 0-443-08058-5

7 6 5 4 3 2 1

Library of Congress Cataloging in Publication Data

Tucker, Harvey M.
  Surgery for phonatory disorders.

    (Monographs in clinical otolaryngology; v. 3)
  Bibliography: p.
  Includes index.
    1. Larynx—Surgery.   2. Voice disorders—
Surgery. I. Title. II. Series. [DNLM:
1. Voice disorders. 2. Larynx—Surgery.
W1 M0567KK v. 3 WV 540 T892s]
RF516.T8   617'.533   81-38539
ISBN 0-443-08058-5   AACR2

To my parents, Bea and Jack Tucker

Preface

In the first half of the present century laryngologists concerned themselves primarily with lifesaving procedures designed to restore airway under emergency conditions or to attempt to remove malignant and nonmalignant conditions from the larynx and upper airway. These surgeons also had to consider infection, blood loss, shock and many other general problems which today have been largely overcome by advances in various aspects of the medical field.

In the last 30 years there has been a concomitant improvement in understanding of laryngeal anatomy and function. Speech pathologists have been urging that the surgeon give greater consideration to preservation and/or restoration of voice after surgical procedures that of necessity must interfere with normal phonation. It seems appropriate, therefore, to attempt to bring together in one volume a number of surgical procedures which have in common the intention to preserve or restore voice function in the face of other laryngeal pathology.

To this end I have tried to include the necessary anatomic, physiologic and surgical considerations to allow the reader to obtain an understanding of the various factors that must be considered when managing patients with surgical voice disorders. In the interest of brevity and in order to make this text useful not only to surgeons but also to other professionals in the speech field, the chapters on anatomy, physiology and diagnosis of voice disorders have been kept short and somewhat simplified. The material presented is accurate, but is by no means as exhaustive as can be found in some of the appropriate references that deal with the individual subjects in greater detail. The surgical chapters are likewise not intended to describe every possible technique that might be used. I have included those techniques that have been most useful and reliable in my hands and those of closely associated colleagues. Nevertheless, I have tried to include a sufficient choice of procedures that the reader will be able to gain some degree of overview of what is available in the field at the time of this writing. I have also tried to specify the advantages and disadvantages of each procedure in the individual management of particular patients.

This book may therefore be regarded as a primer in surgery for phonatory disorders. As is usually the case in surgery of all types, those techniques and procedures that are most satisfactory in one surgeon's hands may not be in another's. The reader is urged to use the bibliography provided as a stepping stone to broader understanding of the many other worthwhile techniques and concepts already in the general literature.

Contents

1 Functional Anatomy and Physiology of the Larynx

INTRODUCTION

To truly appreciate the pathophysiology and appropriate management of various voice disorders, the functional anatomy and normal physiology of the larynx must be thoroughly understood. The various medical professionals who deal with phonatory problems will already have a basic grounding in these subjects, appropriate to their indivdiual disciplines. Therefore, the considerations in this chapter will be approached from a purely functional standpoint, making no attempt to provide a complete treatment of the gross anatomy or the normal physiology in the traditional sense. (For a more detailed discussion of the anatomy and physiology of the larynx, see references 1, 2, and 6.)

ANATOMY[1, 2, 6]

The structural supports for the larynx are provided by several cartilages and one bone (Figs. 1-1 and 1-2). The bony structure is the *hyoid*. This is a sesamoid bone, inasmuch as it has no direct articulation with any other cartilaginous or bony structure and is suspended between the suprahyoid musculature above and strap muscles below. The major cartilage of the larynx is the *thyroid cartilage*. This is a large shield-shaped structure that makes up the layman's "Adam's apple." It provides the anterior and lateral enclosure of the larynx, articulating inferiorly with the *cricoid cartilage*, which is the only complete ring in the upper airway. This articulation takes place through the *cricothyroid joint*, which is a sliding type, allowing both a rocking motion of the thyroid cartilage as well as movement in an anterior and posterior direction. The *epiglottis* differs from the other cartilages of the larynx in that it is not made of hyaline cartilage but is a thin, flexible, elastic fibrocartilage. Like the hyoid bone, it does not articulate directly with any of the other structures in the larynx. It is suspended from the hyoid bone and the inner surface of the thyroid cartilage by appropriate ligaments. The paired *arytenoid cartilages* articulate with the upper posterior surface of the cricoid ring through true synovial *cricoarytenoid joints*. Because of the peculiar shape of the articular surfaces (opposed ellipsoids), this joint permits two types of movement. The first is rotational, allowing the arytenoid to move about a vertical axis. Thus, the vocal processes can be brought towards each other or away from each other as is appropriate, mostly during phonation. The second is a lateral gliding movement that permits the bodies of the arytenoids to slide towards or away from each other. This latter motion is mainly important to airway function. The paired *corniculate* and *cuneiform cartilages* are small and of questionable function in man. These do not articulate with any other structure in the larynx, but serve as "battens" to increase the stiffness and support of the aryepiglottic folds.

With the exception of the articulations between the cricoid cartilage and the arytenoids on the one hand and the thyroid cartilage on the other, the various skeletal structures of the larynx are attached to each other by a series of membranes and ligaments (Figs. 1-2 and 1-3). As noted above, the hyoid bone is suspended between the mandible above and both the laryngotrachael complex and the sternum below. The superior ligamentous attachments of importance include the *hyomandibular ligaments*. These serve as a "check rein" that limits the inferior excursion of the hyoid bone relative to the mandible and thus to the skull. Inferiorly, the hyoid bone is connected to the thyroid cartilage via the *thyrohyoid membrane* and *ligament*. The thyroid cartilage has between it and the cricoid a *cricothyroid membrane* and *liga-*

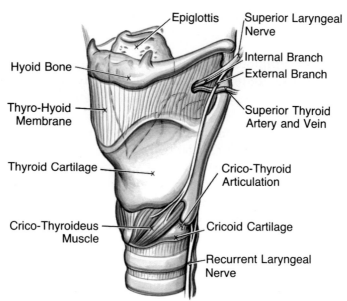

Fig. 1-1 Structural supports of the larynx. The hyoid bone, thyroid cartilage, epiglottic cartilage, cricoid, and first two tracheal rings can be seen. Note the thyrohyoid ligament connecting the hyoid bone and upper border of the thyroid cartilage. It is pierced by the internal branch of the superior laryngeal nerve and by the superior laryngeal artery and vein. The external branch of the superior laryngeal nerve can be seen traversing the thyroid cartilage and innervating the two heads of the cricothyroidius muscle. Note the recurrent laryngeal nerve entering the larynx via two branches in relationship to the inferior cornu of the thyroid cartilage.

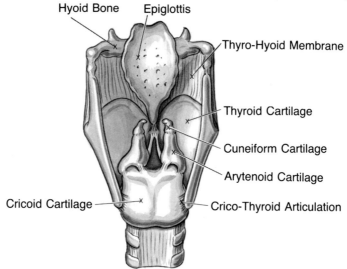

Fig. 1-2 Posterior view of Fig. 1-1. The cricoid lamina is clearly seen, with the arytenoid and cuneiform cartilages resting on its upper border. Perforations in the leaf-shaped epiglottic cartilage can be seen. This view demonstrates the articulation between the inferior cornua of the thyroid cartilage and facets on the lateral surface of the cricoid cartilage. The posterior aspect of the thyrohyoid ligament and the ligamentous structures completing the tracheal rings can be seen.

ment. The epiglottis is suspended from the hyoid bone by the *hyoepiglottic ligament* and from the thyroid cartilage by the *thyroepiglottic ligament,* which is located at the petiole of the epiglottis. The arytenoid cartilages, in addition to the various *cricoarytenoid ligaments* associated with the joint itself, are also connected to the inner surface of the thyroid cartilage by the *vocal* or *thyroarytenoid ligaments* that stretch from the inner surface of the thyroid cartilage to the tips of the vocal processes. These ligaments penetrate the inner perichondrium and cartilage to attach to the undersurface of the outer perichondrium of the hyroid cartilage *(Broyle's ligament).* Internally, a broad, sheetlike membrane stretches from the lateral margins of the epiglottis to the arytenoid and corniculate cartilages. The inferior portion of this forms the *vestibular ligament,* and the major portion is called the *quadrangular membrane.* A fibroelastic membrane stretching from the edges of the true cords inferiorly to insert on the inner surface of the cricoid cartilage is called the *conus elasticus.* The combination of cartilage and bony skeletal elements, together with the various membranes, makes up the gross shape of the larynx.

Most of the internal shape and structure of the larynx is provided by the various intrinsic muscles (Figs. 1-4 A and B). These include the *posterior cricoarytenoideus* (which is the only abductor of the vocal fold), the *lateral cricoarytenoideus, transverse arytenoideus, oblique arytenoideus,* and the *thyroarytenoideus,* which includes in its medial portion the *vocalis.* All of these are paired muscles except for the transverse arytenoid. All but the posterior cricoarytenoideus are adductors and/or tensors of the vocal fold. There are, in addition, paired *cricothyroideus muscles* (Fig. 1-1), which are extrinsic to the larynx, but do have a direct bearing on phonatory function (to be discussed in the next section). In addition, the various *strap muscles* and *pharyngeal constrictors* are also indirectly associated with laryngeal function and phonation.

The soft tissue structures are lined by a continuous *mucosa* composed primarily of respiratory epithelium with goblet cells. The major exception to this occurs on the surface of the vocal folds themselves, which are covered by stratified, nonkeratinizing squamous epithelium. There are no mucous glands on the free edges of the folds. This mucosa is rather loosely attached except where it covers cartilaginous structures, notably the laryngeal surface of the epiglottis and the arytenoid cartilages. There is a potential space filled with loose fibrous tissue between the mucosa and muscularis of the vocal fold. This is referred to as *Reinke's space.*

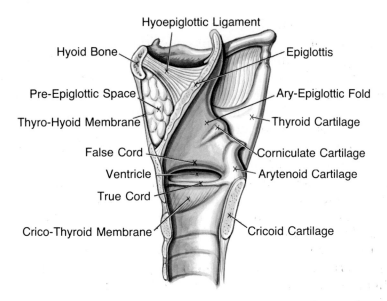

Hyoepiglottic Ligament

Hyoid Bone

Epiglottis

Pre-Epiglottic Space

Ary-Epiglottic Fold

Thyro-Hyoid Membrane

Thyroid Cartilage

False Cord

Corniculate Cartilage

Ventricle

Arytenoid Cartilage

True Cord

Crico-Thyroid Membrane

Cricoid Cartilage

Fig. 1-3   Midline sagittal view of the larynx. The hyoid bone, preepiglottic space, and epiglottic cartilage are demonstrated. Note the hyoepiglottic ligament connecting the inner surface of the hyoid bone to the lingual surface of the epiglottis. This view also demonstrates the signet-ring shape of the cricoid cartilage. Note that the anterior portion of this cartilage is much thinner in its superior-inferior dimension than is the posterior lamina. The greater cornu of the thyroid cartilage is seen with its ligamentous attachment to the greater cornu of the hyoid bone. The left aryepiglottic fold with its supporting cuneiform and corniculate cartilages is demonstrated. The ventricle is also seen.

The continuation of mucosa stretching between the free edge of the epiglottis and the arytenoid cartilage is referred to as the *aryepiglottic fold*, which is supported by the cuneiform and corniculate cartilages. The reflection of the lining mucosa from the aryepiglottic folds to the lateral pharyngeal walls gives rise to the bilateral *pyriform sinuses*, which lie essentially between the arytenoids medially and the inner surface of the thyroid cartilage laterally. The space is open posteriorly into the hypopharynx and anteriorly is pinched off by the reflection of mucosa onto the inner surface of the thyroid cartilage. The aryepiglottic folds separate the upper part of the pyriform from the *laryngeal introitus*. The funnel-shaped structure thus produced, which extends inferiorly to the *false vocal cords*, is sometimes called the *aditus* of the larynx. The reflection of the mucosa over the undersurface of the false cords laterally to the thyroid cartilage and then back over the upper surface of the true cords provides the paired *laryngeal ventricles* (Fig. 1-3). Anteriorly, each of these has a small blind pouch reflecting slightly upward into the substance of the false cord, which is called the *saccule* or *appendix* of the ventricle. Below the free edge of the vocal folds the reflection of mucosa over the conus elasticus provides the *subglottic area*.

The muscles of the larynx receive motor innervation primarily from the *recurrent laryngeal nerves* (Fig. 1-1), which are, in turn, major branches of the *vagus* (Cranial N. X). These nerves also carry sensory impulses from, and supply visceral motor innervation to, the true cords and subglottic structures. The bilateral *superior laryngeal nerves* leave the vagus high in the neck and enter the larynx from above, in company with the *superior laryngeal artery* and *vein* by penetrating the thyrohyoid ligament. Proximal to this point of entry into the larynx the nerve gives off its *external* or *motor branch*, which supplies motor innervation to the cricoarytenoideus muscles. The *internal branch* is mainly sensory, carrying tactile and other sensation from the epiglottis and false cords as far as the surface of the true cords, as well as proprioceptive impulses.

PHYSIOLOGY

The larynx may be regarded as a valve that has three major functions in the human: (1) provision of an airway, (2) protection of the airway, and (3) phonation. Of these, phonatory function is phylogenetically the most recent. The airway is maintained primarily by the skeletal support structures that make up the larynx. The most important of these is the cricoid cartilage, which, as noted above, is the only complete ring. All of the other cartilaginous structures in the larynx and trachea are incomplete posteriorly, the gap being closed by various membranes and muscles. Were it not for the anatomic juxtaposition of the air and food passages crossing at the larynx, a simple tubular structure with ring support would have been sufficient. The need to prevent passage of food and liquid into the trachea and lower respiratory tract has necessitated the development of a closure mechanism. This is provided primarily by the ability of the arytenoid cartilages to traverse medially on the cricoid and come into close apposition to each other. The vocal folds are passively drawn along

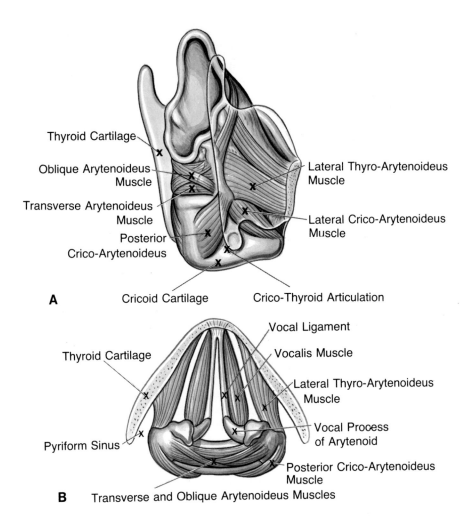

Fig. 1-4 (A and B) *Intrinsic muscles of the larynx.* Note that most of the muscles (with the exception of the vocalis) attach to the lateral or muscular process of the arytenoid cartilages. The interarytenoideus and oblique arytenoideus muscles attach to the medial surfaces of these cartilages. The vocalis muscle and the vocal ligament arise from the vocal process. The origin of the posterior cricoarytenoideus muscle (the only laryngeal abductors) can be seen arising from the posterior thyroid lamina.

with the arytenoids, thus providing glottic closure. However, several other mechanisms are perhaps equally important in this valve action. The extensions of slips of muscle from the thyroarytenoideus into the false cords and along the aryepiglottic folds provide a somewhat weaker but very real closure of these structures during swallowing. Furthermore, the relationship of the thyrotracheal complex to the hyoid bone and thence to the base of the tongue permits an upward movement of the entire larynx during deglutition. A concomitant posterior and downward projection of the posterior third of the tongue passively depresses the epiglottis and aryepiglottic folds down onto the larynx, thus ensuring better closure and deflection of food and water. Liquids, in particular, are directed to one side or the other by the epiglottis and rapidly traverse the pyriform sinuses to bypass the larynx into the hypopharyngeal area. Simultaneously, the reflex opening of the *cricopharyngeus muscle* at the appropriate time during deglutition ensures prompt passage of the bolus of food from the hypopharynx into the upper esophagus.

Another important physiologic factor that helps to prevent aspiration is the relationship of rising supraglottic pressure to opposing subglottic pressure maintained automatically by contraction of the thoracic musculature during swallowing. This is due to the peculiar shape of the false and true cords and their relationship to the ventricles, and plays an important part in the prevention of aspiration. Brunton[3] has shown resistance of the false cords to pressure from below, equaling approximately 30 mmHg. The true cords, on the other hand, will offer relatively little resistance to pressure from below but can resist up to 140-mmHg pressure from above, when approximated. As a result, during swallowing a precise coordination of rising pressure in the hypopharynx against the maintenance of subglottic pressure tends to force the false and true cords more tightly against each other, thus providing even better glottic competence (Fig. 1-5).

Opening of the airway results from the ability of the vocal folds to abduct. This function occurs primarily in response to the action of the posterior cricoarytenoid muscles. These muscles act to draw the vocal processes away from each other by rotating the arytenoid due to muscular pull upon its lateral or muscular process. A small but significant additional increase in cross-sectional airway at the glottis is provided by the thyroarytenoideus muscle. It has been shown that this muscle contracts with inspiration.[4] Although the lateral thyroarytenoideus is the major adductor of the larynx, it must be remembered that for every *agonist* (in this

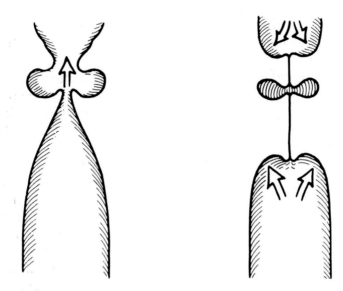

Fig. 1-5 With the cords in tight apposition, rising supraglottic and subglottic pressure tend to force the vocal cords more tightly together, thus sealing the glottis.

case the posterior cricoarytenoid muscles) there must be an *antagonist*. Moreover, when opposed by the pull of the posterior cricoarytenoid muscles, the contraction of the thyroarytenoideus produces a slight increase in the anterior-posterior diameter of the glottic chink at the same time that the abductors are producing a major increase in the transverse diameter.

The remaining adductors of the larynx may be considered to have a secondary respiratory function in that their integrity is important to the maintenance of the cough reflex. Coughing is necessary to respiration not only to clear the airway of secretions but also because it produces a temporary increase in intraalveolar pressure, thus better expanding the small air sacs and improving oxygen transport across the blood-lung barrier, especially in patients with emphysema.

Phylogenetically, the most recent function of the larynx is phonation. This activity also requires intact valvular function. It is now widely accepted that the aerodynamic theory of sound production is correct and that the older, neurochronaxic theory of Husson should be discarded.[5] The aerodynamic theory proposes that sound production requires adduction of the vocal cords to a position close to the midline. With certain variations, depending on the type of attack, the sequence of events thereafter is as follows:

Contraction of the expiratory muscles produces a rise in subglottic air pressure. This results in a rapid escape of air between the nearly apposed vocal folds. Because of Bernoulli's effect, this rapid escape of air through a narrow but partially mobile tube produces a medial displacement of the free edges of the vocal folds. Since they are very close to each other at this point in time they are immediately brought into contact, thus stopping the escape of air. There follows immediately a rise in subglottic pressure, which, when it reaches a sufficient magnitude, drives the vocal folds apart, thus beginning a new escape of air and cycling the entire process over and over again. It is the escape of small puffs of air that produces the vibratory phenomenon interpreted by the listener as sound. The intrinsic muscles of the free edge of the vocal fold, notably the vocalis, modify the pitch and quality of this sound by changing the shape and mass of the free edges of the vocal fold and also by changing the tension between the arytenoid cartilages and the inner surface of the thyroid cartilage. This is achieved not only by contraction of the various phonatory muscles but also by increasing opposition to adduction by the antagonist posterior cricoarytenoid (abductor) muscles. The resulting lengthening of the vocal folds (which at first thought might suggest a deepening of the voice) is more than overcome by the concomitant increase in tension and thinning of the free edges of the vocal folds. Thus pitch is raised. Decrease in pitch is achieved by reversing the process just described. Near the upper extreme of pitch capability, the cricothyroideus muscles will also come into play. Their contraction results in a further increase in tension of the vocal folds because of rotation of the cricoid cartilage posteriorly relative to the thyroid cartilage, thus increasing the distance between the anterior commissure and the arytenoids.

This brief description suggests that sound production is primarily a passive action so far as the vocal cords are concerned. Although this is basically true, the modification of sound in terms of pitch, vocal quality, and loudness is not a passive action, but represents the complicated interaction of the thoracic and subglottic musculature, the intrinsic and extrinsic muscles of the larynx and, to an even greater extent, the shaping, resonance and other factors imposed by the upper airway and nasal passages.

REFERENCES

1. Gray, H.: The anatomy of the human body. Philadelphia: Lea and Febiger, 1973.
2. Hast, M.: Anatomy of the larynx, Chap. 4. In English, G.M. (ed.): Otolaryngology, vol. 3. Hagerstown: Harper & Row, 1978.
3. Brunton, T.L. & Cash, T.: The valvular action of the larynx. J. Anat. Physiol., 17:363, 1883.
4. Suzuki, M., Kirchner, J.A. & Murakami, Y.: The cricothyroid as a respiratory muscle. Ann. Otol. Rhinol. Laryngol., 79:1, 1970.
5. Husson, R.: Etude des phenomenes physiologiques et acoustiques fondamentaux de la voix chantee. These Fac Sc, Paris, 1950.
6. Sasaki, C.T.: Physiology of the larynx, Chap. 7. In English, G.M. (ed.): Otolaryngology, vol. 3. Hagerstown: Harper & Row, 1977.

2 Diagnosis and Analysis of Phonatory Disorders

INTRODUCTION

Depending upon the condition or disease entity responsible, interference with vocal communication can manifest itself in many ways. The patient who has sustained such interference with his ability to produce sound and thus to communicate may suffer any degree of disability, even including complete aphonia. Since appropriate management will depend greatly on the accurate evaluation of the pathophysiologic condition that has given rise to the observed interference with phonation, careful diagnostic evaluation is essential. The approach to such a problem should, therefore, follow the same logical sequence that the diagnosis of any medical complaint requires.

HISTORY

A careful history will often make the difference between a correct diagnosis and the inability to make one. Such information as the time of onset, periodicity, degree of severity, varying effect, and the patient's own impression as to what is the cause of his disorder may be very helpful. A careful drug and toxic history can be important, since many phonatory disorders will be found to be related to changes in hormonal balance, to the use of birth control pills, to exposure to noxious fumes or materials to which the individual happens to be allergic, and so forth. An attempt should be made to assess the patient's emotional and psychosocial status during history taking. The harried mother of small children may find that a great deal of her phonatory difficulty is related to her need to raise her voice to get their attention or to be constantly talking to children in the back seat of a station wagon while she sits in the front, while the busy executive may notice that his difficulty is related to the need to speak under stressful circumstances to moderate-sized groups of people without the assistance of a microphone. The health professional doing this assessment must remember that whereas many individuals may be able to tolerate some of these situational stresses without difficulty, others cannot. Although this text does not permit a detailed discussion of history taking, it is hoped that the reader will appreciate the need for all pertinent background information that can be obtained.

PHYSICAL EXAMINATION

No patient with a disorder of phonation should be considered for treatment without having had a thorough otolaryngologic examination. It should be obvious that mechanical or physiologic causes for changes in voice must be ruled out before such supportive measures as speech therapy or voice rest are undertaken. The otolaryngologist needs to do a thorough examination, giving attention not only to the larynx and vocal cords, but also to the remainder of the upper aerodigestive tract and the entire head and neck. Such adjacent structures as the thyroid gland may need careful assessment in some cases, while a previously undetected mass in the lateral neck might lead to careful inspection of hidden areas within the larynx where a primary malignancy might lurk. In short, the tenet that a voice change of 2 weeks' duration or greater requires careful otolaryngologic assessment still holds true. In selected cases, findings either in the history or the otolaryngologic examination may suggest that a more thorough general physical examination be undertaken as well. Certain endocrine disorders may manifest themselves early in the larynx, as, for example, in hypothyroidism. Many central nervous system disorders will involve voice change and a careful physical examination may lead the physician to suggest a neurologic evaluation as well, in these cases.

X-RAY EVALUATION

Most patients with voice disorders will have some finding on physical examination or history that will direct the attention of the evaluating physician to appropriate systems. If the diagnosis is obvious, (e.g., a case of vocal nodules) no special x-ray evaluation will be needed other than a chest x-ray, which is usually required before an anesthetic can be administered if surgery is recommended. Most morphologic changes in the larynx are detectable by indirect mirror examination. However, if a patient is found to have unilateral vocal cord paralysis of undetermined etiology, a very careful x-ray evaluation, including chest films, cine barium swallow, and tomograms of the base of the skull may be needed. On occasion, studies such as contrast laryngogram or xeroradiography may be of value. These latter studies are more often confirmatory or give greater weight to a possible diagnosis than they are definitive by themselves. Although a cine barium swallow is not directed precisely at the larynx, it may show evidence of dyssynergia or other abnormality in swallowing, which would suggest the possibility of central nervous system disorders, such as amyotrophic lateral sclerosis. Skull x-rays may show areas of tumor involvement of the base of the skull or erosion or enlargement of the various foramena that provide exit for important cranial nerves involved in speech production.

VOICE ASSESSMENT[1]

"Doctor, I am hoarse" will be the chief complaint of most patients with a voice change. This self-diagnosis is incorrect in a surprising number of patients, however. The patient really means that there has been some change in the quality, loudness, pitch, or clarity of the voice, detected either by the patient himself or by his associates. Almost any of the above-mentioned voice changes will usually be interpreted as "hoarseness." It is important, therefore, that the person assessing such "hoarseness" be able to distinguish between the various deviations from customary voice that may lead the patient to seek medical advice.

Such deviations perceived by the listener may be due to alterations in three variables: loudness, quality, and pitch. With practice and careful listening, the professional charged with evaluating this disorder may be able to discern, with reasonable accuracy, the probable physiologic source, occasionally the general nature of the pathologic condition, and sometimes the best initial approach to therapy, simply by listening to the voice. Needless to say, this impression will have to be confirmed by direct observation, biopsy, and/or other measures in every case.

1. *Disorders of loudness.* Most disorders of loudness will stem from disability in one of three general areas. These include inadequate control of air flow, inability to approximate the vocal cords, and/or hearing loss. The first and third of these may be due to correctable problems but are really not within the purview of this text. Suffice it to say that patients who have poor motor control of the diaphragm and intercostal muscles often have a very weak voice because they cannot produce sufficient air flow to increase volume. On the other hand, the patient with conductive hearing deficit will often speak in a soft voice because his voice sounds loud to him. The patient with sensorineural hearing loss, as exemplified by an elderly individual with presbycusis, will often speak in a very loud voice for the converse reason. Inability to approximate the vocal folds for whatever reason will result in a weak voice because of rapid air escape and decreased vibration produced at the level of the vocal folds. Occasionally, a disorder of loudness will be intermittent, suggesting vocal fatigue. Such diseases as myasthenia gravis may present in this fashion, even though the patient has fairly normal volume and pitch control at other times.

2. *Disorders of pitch.* Any organic or neurologic pathology that produces a change or interference with vocal fold thickness, tension, cross-sectional mass, or minute control of the folds themselves may result in an alteration in pitch level. Hormonal changes, as in the menstrual cycle or in thyroid dysfunction, can produce pitch control difficulties that are not always easily accounted for by directly observing the vocal folds themselves. More often, changes in pitch may be habitual or result from normal maturational processes in both boys and girls.

3. *Disorders of vocal quality.* Some 66 different words have been used in the literature to describe changes in vocal quality. If such terms as denasality, excess nasal resonance, and so forth (all of which are changes in quality that result from problems outside the larynx), are eliminated from consideration, only *breathiness,*

harshness, roughness, and *diplophonia* are left as useful descriptive terms. Any or all of these may be considered variants of hoarseness. Diplophonia, which may be due to either paralysis or paresis of the superior laryngeal or recurrent laryngeal nerves, will often be interpreted by the listener as "roughness" or "hoarseness" simply because the human ear cannot always distinguish between two pitches that vary from each other only by a few Hertz. Most lesions that result in disorders of vocal quality will be discernible by indirect or direct laryngeal examination, whether they are secondary to disorders of cord mobility or to mass lesions involving the vibratory surfaces of the cords. A few of these, however, are quite evanescent, and careful examination under proper circumstances is required to demonstrate them. Such conditions as spasmodic dysphonia and dysphonia plica ventricularis may present apparently normal larynges to mirror examination, unless the observer is able to detect the small but significant changes in mobility. Spasmodic dysphonia, for example, will usually demonstrate a normal appearing larynx with normal abduction and adduction of the vocal cords, except that during phonation tremor and choked voice are produced because of the effort of both cords to cross the midline simultaneously. Dysphonia plica ventricularis, on the other hand, requires observation that the false cords make contact with each other during phonation before the true cords do. In the usual examination circumstances, when the tongue is being pulled forward, this condition may be hard to demonstrate because of the unusual position. In order to prove the diagnosis, it is often necessary to use either motion picture contrast studies in an anterior-posterior projection or a flexible fiberoptic instrument introduced through the nose so that the position of the epiglottis and base of tongue is not disrupted.

PATIENT EDUCATION

Once a diagnosis has been arrived at or at least is strongly suspected, the patient should be instructed carefully in the nature of his or her disorder, the possibilities for appropriate therapy, and should be made to understand what reasonable expectations exist for cure. For example, the patient with simple vocal polyps enjoys a high probability that a more or less normal voice can be restored either through appropriate speech therapy, the removal of irritants such as smoking or allergy, and/or in certain cases surgical removal by laryngoscopy. If, on the other hand, the patient is a professional soprano with small vocal nodules interfering with her highest pitch range, it is imperative that she understand that in spite of all efforts, including careful surgical management, it may never be possible to restore her voice to what it was before her problem began. In short, the patient, the speech pathologist, and the physician must have a common and realistic expectation of what can be achieved and an accurate understanding of the disease entity to be treated. Only in this fashion can the patient take an active part in management of the disorder. Without such informed cooperation, many times the best efforts of the professionals treating the patient will be doomed to failure. The psychological benefits of a thorough understanding of one's problem and what can be achieved to correct it cannot be overestimated.

REFERENCE

1. Perkins, W.H.: Mechanisms of vocal abuse. In Weinberg, B. (ed.): Transcripts of the 7th Symposium on Care of the Professional Voice. Part II. New York: The Voice Foundation, 1978.

3 Management of Mass Lesions of the Larynx

INTRODUCTION

Since phonatory function depends on the ability of the vocal cords to vibrate freely, any mass lesion involving either the edge of the vocal cord or interfering with its vibratory capacity will result in a change in this function. Although the many lesions that will be considered in this chapter differ from each other in such significant parameters as etiology, pathophysiology, and prognosis, they have in common such interference with the passive vibratory function of the cords noted above. Because of this, certain general principles of surgical management can be applied to them and they can therefore be considered jointly. Almost without exception, such lesions are visible on physical examination with the laryngeal mirror and only occasionally require direct laryngoscopy for diagnosis. In any event, proper management for each of these lesions will necessitate direct laryngoscopy either in a diagnostic capacity or more frequently for appropriate management. Mastery of available techniques for endolaryngeal diagnosis and surgical management through the laryngoscope is therefore a cornerstone of laryngologic practice.

DIRECT LARYNGOSCOPY

Direct laryngoscopy may be performed quite satisfactorily under local anesthesia for most diagnostic and many therapeutic needs. However, with the advent of safe, effective general anesthestic techniques, the frequency with which local anesthesia is used has been decreasing in most hands. Nevertheless, it remains important that the laryngologist be able to administer effective, safe local anesthetic in many cases.

Local Anesthesia

The technique to be described is that used by the author and is modified from the general technique described by Chevalier Jackson.[1] Pontocaine (tetracaine), 0.5 percent is used. This drug is at the same time the most effective and most toxic of the "caine" drugs after cocaine itself. It is effective, however, in dilute solution and therefore can be used safely, provided it is applied accurately and the total dose used at any one time does not exceed the maximal recommended dose of 80 mg.[2] The author does not exceed 8 ml of 0.5 percent solution so that not more than half the recommended dose is used in any individual case. Experience in over a thousand cases using this technique has failed to reveal a single true toxic reaction.

The patient is placed in a sitting position and asked to stick out his tongue (Fig. 3-1) and to hold it in extension using his right hand. The surgeon stands in front of the patient with a headlight or mirror and proceeds as follows: the anesthetic solution is drawn up in a control syringe attached to a flexible blunt cannula. The cannula is curved at its distal end to approximately 90 degrees (Fig. 3-2). A maximum of 0.5 to 1.0 ml of solution is drawn up. The laryngeal mirror is held in the examiner's left hand, warmed, and placed in the usual position to visualize the larynx. The cannula is then introduced taking care not to stimulate a gag reflex. When the tip of the cannula can be seen to be pointed directly at the vocal cords the patient is asked to inspire and at that instant the entire bolus of solution is ejected into the larynx between the vocal cords (Fig. 3-3). If the application is completely successful, there will be an immediate coughing reaction which will serve both to produce an aerosol of the solution and to spread it around the supraglottic structures at the same time. In patients whose larynges are easily visualized and in whom the solution can be placed accurately on the first try, a single such instillation is often adequate for direct

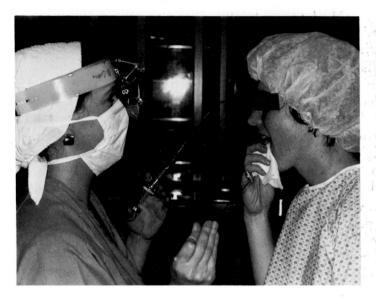

Fig. 3-1   Patient is asked to extend the tongue and to hold it in this position using the right hand.

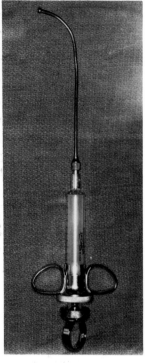

Fig. 3-2   Syringe and cannula for instillation of topical anesthesia in laryngoscopy.

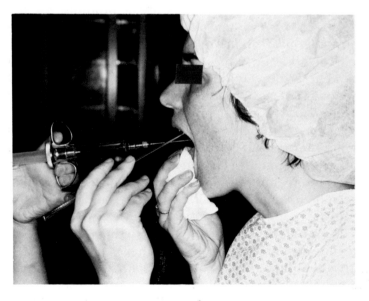

Fig. 3-3   Topical anesthetic is instilled directly between the vocal cords, while simultaneously observing them with a laryngeal mirror.

laryngoscopy. Most cases require that the applications be repeated until 6 or 8 ml have been used. The patient is probably ready for laryngoscopy when there is no cough reflex for at least a few seconds after a significant amount of solution has been instilled. This indicates that the supraglottic, glottic, and subglottic structures are suitably anesthetized.

Patients may be premedicated with 200 mg of Nembutol, orally approximately 1 hour, and Demerol, 50 to 75 mg, and Vistaril, 25 to 50 mg, injected IM approximately 20 to 30 minutes before the anticipated procedure. It has been the author's experience, however, that with good rapport and careful selection of patients for local anesthesia, no premedication, other than 0.2 mg of atropine to minimize secretions, is preferable. Although it is not the subject of this chapter, it should be noted that the same anesthetic technique has also been used with good results for esophagoscopy and bronchoscopy.

General Anesthesia

As noted above, it is becoming more popular to employ general anesthesia for all endoscopic procedures, particularly those that require extended surgical manipulation or a suspension laryngoscope. The standard techniques are a problem for the otolaryngologist, since an endotracheal tube is required. It is possible to perform adequate endoscopy with a small endotracheal tube in place. To this end, it is important to use the smallest possible tube that will provide life support for the patient throughout the length of the procedure. In most cases this will be a standard endotracheal tube with an inside diameter of 5.0 to 5.5 mm. Relaxation is usually desirable, except where spontaneous movement of the vocal cords must be assessed. The technique most commonly used is light inhalation anesthesia coupled with a paralytic agent. This technique has an advantage in that the patient's mouth can be opened to its widest capacity and any motion of the vocal cords avoided during critical manipulations.

It is often desirable to examine the larynx or even work within it without the interference of an endotracheal tube. For such cases, alternative techniques are available. The first of these is the *apneic technique*. The patient is anesthetized, paralyzed as for intubation, and hyperventilated to raise blood oxygen levels to near saturation. Then, without intubation, the appropriate laryngoscope is introduced and the surgeon allowed to work within the larynx for 1 to 2 minutes. During this time, the anesthesiologist monitors pulse, blood pressure, and the ECG. At the anesthesiologist's request, the laryngoscopist will remove all instruments and allow the patient to be ventilated again, using a mask. With good rapport between anesthesiologist and surgeon, this procedure can be carried out with minimal difficulty in properly selected cases. No significant bleeding should be anticipated, since this might be difficult to control and still allow the anesthesiologist to ventilate the patient as necessary.

The second technique employs a *high-pressure Venturi apparatus*, which can be attached to the open end of the laryngoscope and allows the anesthesiologist to apply a blast of high-pressure oxygen through the relaxed vocal cords. In this fashion, the patient can be ventilated almost continuously throughout the procedure. There is a small risk of rupture of alveoli with this technique, especially in children. It is, nevertheless, a useful method in experienced hands. A third approach is the use of the *Carden tube*.[3] This requires a special endotracheal tube with two narrow channels, one for cuff inflation and the other for the application of anesthetic gases and oxygen. These are attached distally to a short length of cuffed endotracheal tubing. When in place, this allows reasonable control of respiration with minimal interference and with working space for the surgeon. The procedure requires experience in tube placement and suffers because anesthetic gases are blown back into the surgeon's face. Finally, the *mass transfer technique* can be used. The patient is anesthetized and paralyzed, intubated, and hyperventilated using pure oxygen towards the end of the hyperventilation period. A single fine catheter is placed in the posterior commissure and down the trachea, through which oxygen is delivered at high rate of flow. As oxygen is absorbed through the alveoli, it is gradually replaced by the high flow from above. This will permit several minutes working time without the patient being actually ventilated. Carbon dioxide continues to accumulate, since it is not blown off, and can produce problems if the procedure is carried on too long.

The author has come to use the apneic technique almost exclusively. For most applications, this is more than adequate in terms of working time. It is nontraumatic and does not require special equipment. It *does* require that either the anesthesiologist or the otolaryngologist be prepared to intubate the patient promptly, immediately if necessary. For this reason, a small bronchoscope is available on the operating table throughout the procedure in case rapid intubation cannot be achieved in the usual fashion.

Technique of Direct Laryngoscopy

With the patient in a supine position under suitable local or general anesthesia, the head is placed in the so-called "sniffing" position. This may be described as flexion of the neck on the thorax and extension of the head on the neck, and it can be achieved in several ways: (1) a head-holder (assistant) may support the patient's head in this position, as originally described by Chevalier Jackson;[1] (2) the head can be supported on a "donut" or other apparatus in the desired position; or (3) the operator may sit sideways at the head of the table, supporting the patient's head on his own iliac crest, with one leg braced on the floor, then by leaning against the patient, the patient's head can be placed in the desired position and kept there, leaving the operator's hands free for manipulation (Fig. 3-4). The importance of appropriate positioning cannot be stressed too strongly. It is necessary to try to produce as straight a line as possible between the upper alveolar ridge and the introitus of the larynx for maximal visualization and adequate room for manipulation. The appropriate laryngoscope is selected.

In the author's hands, the most commonly used laryngoscope for examination purposes is the Hollinger modification of the Jackson anterior commissure laryngoscope (Fig. 3-5), although a Jackson slide laryngoscope is also sometimes useful. The latter instrument was actually designed for placement of a bronchoscope, but can be very useful for examining the structures around the larynx, particularly the base of the tongue. The laryngoscope is introduced with the dominant hand (right hand in a right-handed surgeon), with the lateral aspect of the laryngoscope placed against the tongue under direct vision. It is then rotated slightly to bring it into the proper position and then transferred to the opposite hand. At this point, the examiner transfers his line of sight from along the side of the laryngoscope to the lumen of the instrument itself. In most cases, the tip of the epiglottis will already be visible, if the laryngoscope has been placed properly (Fig. 3-6). The laryngoscope handle is balanced between the hypothenar eminence and the crotch between the thumb and index finger (Fig. 3-7). This is important for a number of reasons. First, the instrument has been designed to be held in this fashion. When so grasped, it is automatically in the proper position and allows very little leverage to be applied, except in the proper direction (to be discussed below), thus minimizing the possibility of traumatizing the epiglottis or the vocal folds with the tip of the instrument. The free hand is then placed so that the index finger is

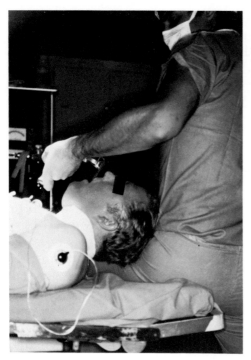

Fig. 3-4 Patient in position for direct laryngoscopy. Note that with head on iliac crest and operator resting on the operating table, it is possible to control the head in the "sniffing position" leaving the right hand free for necessary manipulations.

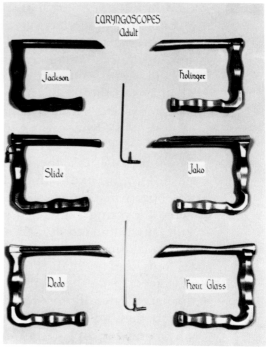

Fig. 3-5 Various laryngoscopes.

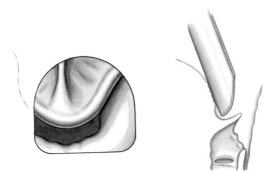

Fig. 3-6 Laryngoscopic view of epiglottis after initial placement of laryngoscope. Position of the laryngoscope is illustrated to the right.

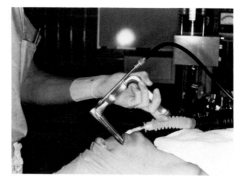

Fig. 3-7 Proper balance of laryngoscope in left hand, resting between the hypothenar eminence and the crotch between the thumb and index finger.

against the upper teeth and the thumb is on the lower margin of the opening of the laryngoscope. The left hand is used to support and advance the 'scope, and the right hand is used to guide it. In this fashion, the epiglottis and valleculae can be examined along with the supraglottic structures. The laryngoscope is then relaxed slightly and the tip of it allowed to pick up the free edge of the epiglottis. The laryngoscope is carefully advanced a few millimeters and again positioned by displacing it towards the patient's feet (Fig. 3-8). The concept that the instrument is advanced as a unit, such that the weight of the patient is borne along the posterior third of the tongue, is extremely important. If the laryngoscope is manipulated as described above and care is taken to avoid "levering", and if the entire instrument is advanced as a unit, any trauma to the larynx will be minimized. At this point in the procedure, it is possible to observe the false cords, aryepiglottic folds, and arytenoids (Fig. 3-9). The laryngoscope may now be advanced to the level of the glottis or, as the examiner prefers, displaced laterally to examine the two pyriform sinuses. In any event, the larynx is further exposed by carefully and slowly advancing the tip of the laryngoscope to slightly displace the false cords, thus providing a good view of the true vocal folds (Fig. 3-10).

Various instruments and suction tips may now be used to examine, palpate and, if necessary, manipulate the vocal folds themselves or any lesions related to them (Fig. 3-11). The scope of this treatise does not permit a detailed discussion of all the instruments available for laryngoscopy. The common instruments are various sized cup forceps (upbiting, straight, and angulated) and small alligator forceps. These latter are used to grasp lesions, and the former are used to both grasp and remove lesions.

A general comment can be made regarding the use of cup forceps for removing lesions that involve the superficial mucosa of the larynx and of the vocal cord in particular. When Reinke's space is not traversed by the lesion (which is the usual situation, with the possible exception of malignancies), it is better to strip the lesion away rather than to "bite" it off. This can be done with minimum trauma if the following technical steps are followed: The laryngoscope is rotated slightly so that the lip is towards the side of the lesion, thus fixing the vocal cord at its tip and minimizing any movement of the lesion (Fig. 3-12). A small upbiting cup forceps is introduced and the lesion is grasped gently, but not so firmly as to cut through its attachment (Fig. 3-13). If the forceps is quickly and sharply advanced along the long axis of the

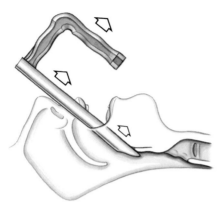
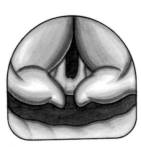
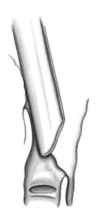

Fig. 3-8 Proper positioning of the laryngoscope. Note that further exposure of the larynx is obtained by advancing the entire instrument towards the patient's feet and the ceiling rather than by angulation or "levering" against the upper teeth.

Fig. 3-9 Initial view of aryepiglottic folds, false cords, and arytenoid cartilages after proper placement of the laryngoscope.

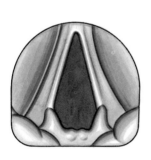
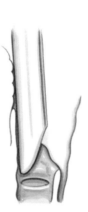
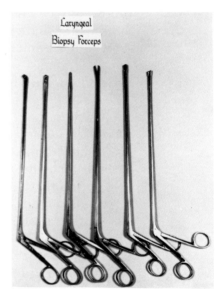

Fig. 3-10 Final laryngoscopic view of the true vocal cords.

Fig. 3-11 Various laryngeal forceps.

trachea and then immediately drawn back in a single in and out motion, the mucosa at the point of attachment of the lesion will tear neatly away through Reinke's space leaving a smooth, denuded vocal cord (Fig. 3-14). If small shreds of torn mucosa are left, these can be gently removed with the cup forceps. This technique is useful for polyps, nodules, as well as some papillomata of the vocal cord, and may also be used in attempts to

"strip" the vocal cord for leukoplakia and other surface phe-
nomena. In fact, when a benign-looking lesion resists removal
in this fashion, because of invasion through Reinke's space into
the muscular portion of the vocal cord and is so adherent that it
must be bitten off, this often suggests malignancy.

Technique of Suspension Microlaryngoscopy

Although the techniques for direct laryngoscopy described
above are adequate for most lesions encountered by the otolaryngologist, the advent of the suspension laryngoscope, coupled with
microsurgical instruments and the operating microscope, has revolutionized endolaryngeal surgery. Whereas the experienced surgeon can achieve satisfactory results with a nonmicroscopic
technique in most cases, such a level of skill requires constant
practice and a very large training experience. On the other hand,
almost any competent surgeon can achieve equal or superior results with somewhat less experience, using suspension laryngoscopy and the microscope.

It is almost always necessary to perform suspension microlaryngoscopy under general anesthesia with a small tube in place.
The types of laryngoscopes used vary greatly and can include the
standard Jackson laryngoscopes. However, both the Jako and
Dedo laryngoscopes have been designed for better exposure of
the larynx for microsurgical procedures (Fig. 3-15A and B). When
suitable anesthesia has been obtained, the laryngoscope is inserted exactly as described for direct laryngoscopy. Once it has
been positioned as desired, a suspension apparatus is attached.
The author prefers the Lewy arm for this purpose and rests the
distal end on a Mayo stand appropriately placed over the patient's
chest (Fig. 3-16). This apparatus is adjusted to the proper tension,
and the operating microscope is then brought into position. The
fine microsurgical instruments, including scissors, spatulae, and
various types of knives, as well as cup forceps and alligator forceps, permit meticulous removal of small lesions with minimal
damage to surrounding structures (Fig. 3-17A-C). The basic principles, however, remain exactly the same; that is, lesions limited
to the mucosa are removed by excising the mucous membrane
through Reinke's space, trying to leave the underlying muscularis
and vocal ligament as little traumatized as possible. As a general
rule, one avoids removing mucosa from both sides of the anterior
commissure at a single procedure since, when this is done, web
formation may result.

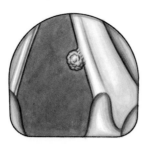

Fig. 3-12 Proper positioning of laryngoscope for removal of vocal cord lesion. Note that the tip of the scope has been used to displace the false cord on the right and to fix the true cord with the lesion on it in full view.

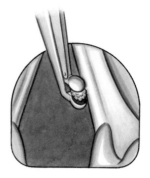

Fig. 3-13 The lesion is grasped with the angulated cup forceps.

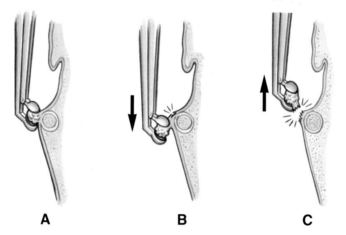

A   B   C

Fig. 3-14 Proper avulsion/stripping technique for removal of pedunculated lesions of the vocal cord. (A) The lesion is grasped firmly with a cup forceps but not "bitten" off. (B) The forceps is displaced along the long axis of the trachea with a sharp in-and-out motion. This results in an initial tear along the upper surface of the vocal cord adjacent to the base of the lesion. (C) With a single motion, the forceps is then retracted along the long axis of the trachea thus completing the tear along the lower surface of the vocal cord.

Laser Surgery of the Larynx

The surgical CO_2 laser has significantly improved the ability of the laryngeal surgeon to work within a confined space.[4-6] This instrument permits meticulous destruction or removal of tissues within the larynx with virtually no damage to adjacent tissues.

Because of the wavelength of the coherent light being used, the distance from total tissue destruction to normal cells is approximately 60μ. Since very little eschar and almost no edema results, lesions removed in this fashion heal very promptly. No delay is necessary while partially damaged tissue goes on to necrosis and slough. In addition, since the instrument that does the cutting is actually a beam of light, precious operating space through the narrow laryngoscope is conserved so that other instruments can be used for retraction and stabilization while the beam is in use. Specialized metal instruments, such as mirrors, suction retractors, and protectors (Fig. 3-18), are needed for certain applications. In general, any lesion that can be exposed in direct line of sight through a suspension laryngoscope, or which can be seen in this configuration reflected in a metal mirror, can be destroyed or removed accurately using the CO_2 laser.

It is tempting to conclude that this very useful instrument will supplant standard microsurgical or laryngoscopic techniques. This is unlikely for a number of reasons, however. To begin with, the instrumentation necessary for laser surgery is quite expensive and, in the present state of the art, fairly cumbersome. It seems unlikely that the laryngologist that does such surgery only on occasion will be able to justify the expense involved. For this reason, the laser will probably be limited to fairly large institutions in which several practicing laryngologists will make use of it. Secondly, this instrument requires special training to qualify otherwise experienced laryngologists to use it. Until more centers are available, which either include laser surgery in the training program of new residents or make short courses in laser surgery available to practicing otolaryngologists, it will be difficult to obtain the necessary skills. Third and most important, there are only a limited number of lesions in which the laser provides a *real* advantage over properly used microsurgical techniques. Most noteworthy among these is laryngeal papillomatosis (which will be discussed in detail below). Other lesions that are managed with greater ease and perhaps better success with the laser include contact ulcers, intubation granulomata, and small vascular lesions of the larynx. The laser permits coagulation of vessels up

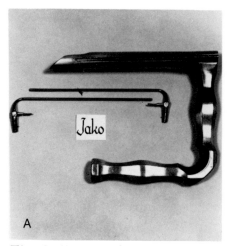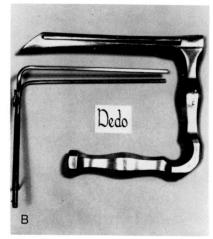

Fig. 3-15 (A) Jako suspension laryngoscope. (B) Dedo suspension laryngoscope.

to 0.5 mm in diameter with virtually no bleeding. Thus, such lesions as lymphangiomas, hemangiomas, and neuromas of the larynx can be managed very nicely with this instrument. The laser can be very helpful in the management of such common laryngologic lesions as nodules and polyps, but is certainly not essential. One other area in which the laser may prove to be very important in the near future is the management of leukoplakia, hyperkeratosis with atypia, carcinoma in situ, and even certain early carcinomas of the true vocal cord, which are presently managed either by radiation or by gross surgical excision.[6]

Currently available CO_2 lasers are all quite similar. Most of them are mounted on an operating microscope and a "joy-stick" is used to manipulate the direction of the beam (Fig. 3-19). An aiming system, employing a marker light, is also common to the existing instruments. The light is seen on the surface of the larynx either in real or virtual image and, when properly aimed, the laser beam will strike this point. The amount of tissue destruction is controlled by setting the power and time of exposure to suitable levels.

It is imperative that certain precautions be taken during laser surgery. First, the endotracheal tube used must be wrapped with a reflecting aluminum or silver tape to prevent the laser beam from burning through the plastic and perhaps causing a flash fire, if oxygen at high flow within the tube is encountered (Fig. 3-20). Secondly, neurosurgical patties soaked in saline are placed around the tube below the vocal cords so that any stray beam that misses the edge of the soft tissue will not strike the distal tracheal wall or the tube. Third, the patient's eyes are carefully covered with wet eyepads and then taped into position. Since water absorbs the laser beam, any wet substance will protect adjacent tissues. Finally, all personnel in the operating room should be wearing eye protection, either glasses or goggles, in case there should be stray reflection of the beam. Needless to say, explosive anesthetic gases are never used in laser surgery.

General Considerations

Regardless of the instrument used, direct laryngoscopic techniques have certain general considerations in common. The patient must understand that whatever technique is used and regardless of the quality of the voice before surgery, there will be a period of hoarseness which may vary from several hours to as much as 2 or 3 months after surgery. It is equally important to tape record the voice of any patient who is to undergo endolaryngeal surgery. This is not only for the protection of the surgeon from a medical/legal standpoint (such as one would achieve with preoperative photographs before cosmetic surgery) but also to assist the speech professional in assessing voice disorders or assisting the patient to recover good vocal function afterwards. It cannot be stressed too strongly that a speech pathologist should be in consultation on all patients who are to undergo laryngeal surgery. This is particularly important when it is known that there will be some permanent or semipermanent effect on the voice. It will be extremely helpful, if not essential, to the speech pathologist that he or she see the patient for at least one visit before surgery is undertaken.

In the past, it was often customary to require that patients who have had endolaryngeal surgery undertake complete voice rest for a period of as much as 2 weeks from the time of surgery. More recently, many surgeons have felt that this was not only excessive but unrealistic. At present, the author requires 48 hours of absolute voice rest following surgery that involves stripping or other trauma to the phonatory surfaces of the true vocal cords, followed by a period of minimal voice use for about 2 weeks. The patient is instructed, during this period, to avoid all vocal stress. This includes such things as speaking in public, trying to talk over background noise, such as at a cocktail party or in a bar, trying to talk to children in the backseat while sitting in the front seat of an automobile, and so forth. As a general rule of thumb, we urge our patients not to try to talk to anyone that they could not touch while

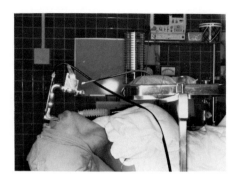

Fig. 3-16 Suspension laryngo-scope in position using Mayo stand for support.

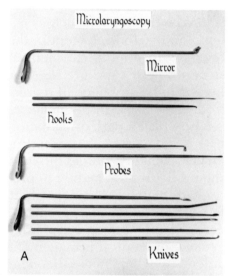

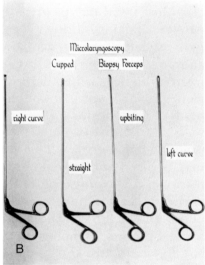

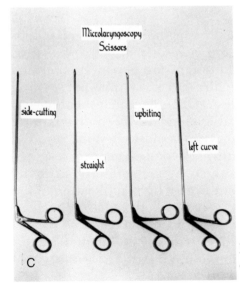

Fig. 3-17 (A–C) Microlaryngos-copy instruments.

doing so. The speech therapist provides training in proper vocal hygiene during this healing period. The patient is seen at roughly 2-week intervals until such time as it is clear that the surgical site is completely healed and/or the voice has returned essentially to normal.

MANAGEMENT OF SPECIFIC LESIONS

Polyps (Fig. 3-21)

Most vocal polyps are the result of local trauma, such as excessive smoking, allergy, vocal abuse, and so forth. Except in the most advanced stages, many will regress with appropriate medical and voice therapy. Cessation of smoking or of exposure to other toxic influences is mandatory if there is to be any hope of regression. Proper vocal hygiene is the other mainstay in the management of these lesions. If allergy is felt to play a part, consultation with an allergist or management by the otolaryngologist appropriate to the allergy will be helpful. Occasionally, steroid inhalers may be used but these attempts should be limited mainly to professionals who must perform or get through a relatively short period of vocal stress and can follow this with an appropriate period of voice rest. We have preferred the Decadron Respihaler for this purpose. When a suitable course of medical management has been undertaken and has failed, or when it has become apparent that the patient is unwilling or unable to cooperate in such management, consideration must be given to surgical removal of the polyps.

From a clinical standpoint, three general types of polyps occur: *pedunculated, fusiform,* and *generalized polypoid degeneration* (Fig. 3-22). Pedunculated polyps are generally managed most successfully with microsurgical excision, preserving maximum adjacent normal mucosa. Once complete healing has ensued and training in good vocal hygiene has been given, these usually do not recur. The fusiform type is most often the result of acute vocal trauma, such as shouting at a football game or a severe bout of coughing. These are managed by meticulously stripping the involved area, and may benefit from a light application of the laser to the remaining mucosa to "spot weld" the adjacent mucosa to the underlying muscular surface. Although it cannot be proved histologically, this procedure helps to partially obliterate Reinke's space and, perhaps, in this fashion minimizes the possibility that

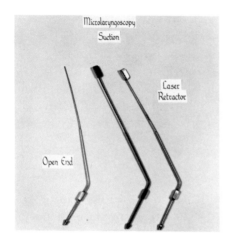

Fig. 3-18 Suction retractors for laser surgery. The angulated apparatus at the tip of the suction is used to displace and protect the adjacent vocal cord during lasering.

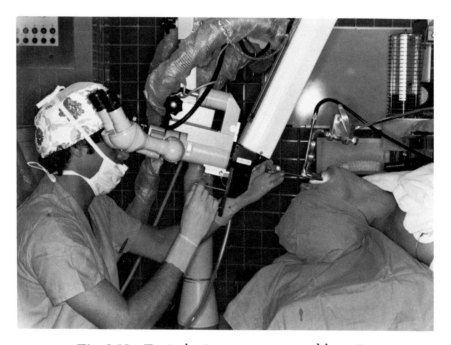

Fig. 3-19 Typical microscope-mounted laser in use.

edema fluid will again accumulate. Diffuse polypoid change is most often an endstage condition resulting from prolonged laryngeal abuse and/or allergy and these patients rarely respond to nonsurgical management. Nevertheless, before surgery is undertaken, every effort should be made to get the patient to stop smoking, and intensive training in vocal hygiene should be begun so that after surgical stripping has been undertaken the best possibility of nonrecurrence of the conditions that produced the polypoid change in the first place can be expected. We have found the laser very useful in the careful removal of these lesions, although they can certainly be managed satisfactorily with microsurgical technique.

Reinke's Edema

This condition is hard to differentiate from a fusiform or diffuse type polyp and probably represents an early state in polyp formation. If the irritant that has produced the edema is not reversed, it probably will go on to a frank polyp. Patients who persist in producing this type of edema should be considered for evaluation of thyroid status, since myxedema of the larynx is not uncommonly present when other symptoms of hypothyroidism are as yet not manifest. An intensive period of nonsurgical management, including good vocal hygiene, should be attempted in every such case since most of them will resolve if treated appropriately. In the rare persistent or recurrent case a very superficial lasering may be helpful in preventing recurrence for the same reason stated in the paragraph above.

Vocal Nodules

To fully understand the management of vocal nodules requires careful definitions of terms. Although many pathologists feel that nodules are nothing more than endstage vocal polyps, I believe that such a view represents a misunderstanding of the pathophysiology of the lesion. It is important to differentiate between the *clinical* and the *pathologic* diagnosis of vocal nodule. The former is reserved for small sessile lesions limited to the junction of the anterior and middle thirds of the vocal cord, usually bilateral, and often associated with a history of vocal abuse (Fig. 3-23A). These lesions may be hemorrhagic, but more often are pale, whitish, and may or may not be associated with localized edema.

The *pathologic* diagnosis of nodule, however, specifically

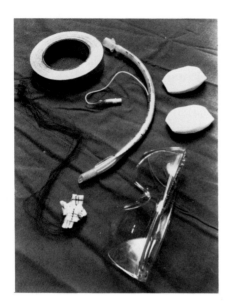

Fig. 3-20 Safety equipment for use in laser surgery. Note the endotracheal tube wrapped with silver tape proximal to the balloon.

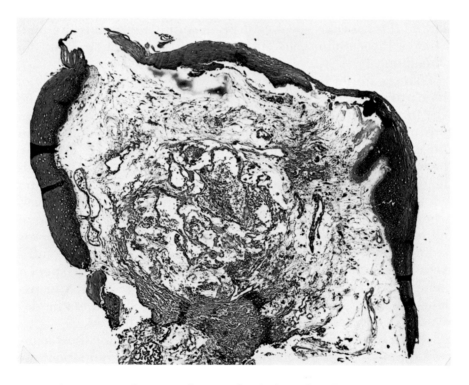

Fig. 3-21 Hemorrhagic and myxoid vocal cord polyp. Note the loose myxoid stroma with multiple small vascular spaces surrounded by essentially normal vocal cord mucosa.

refers to a localization of fibrous or scar tissue in the submucosal area of the vocal cord (Fig. 3-24). This usually has intact, but somewhat hypertrophied mucosa on its surface. If one accepts this definition, it becomes clear that vocal hygiene and medical management of nodules cannot logically play any successful part in eradicating them. Clearly, if the vocal nodule is a mass of scar tissue, voice rest will not cause it to disappear. Nevertheless, it is appropriate to treat all patients who appear with a *clinical* diagnosis of vocal nodules with speech therapy and other medical measures for a period of perhaps as much as 6 weeks because not every lesion that is clinically a vocal nodule is actually an end-stage fibrous lesion. Not infrequently, one of the two "kissing" lesions that appear to be vocal nodules is actually a small polyp resulting from the irritation produced by the true nodule on the other vocal cord. In such cases, one of the two "nodules" will seem to disappear with good vocal hygiene. Secondly, polyps can and do occur at this point on the vocal cord and may even represent early stages of what eventually will become true fibrous nodules. Such a lesion occurs at the junction of the anterior and middle thirds of the vocal cord because this represents the midpoint of the membranous cord, which is the functional unit for phonation.

The posterior third of the cord, which is made up entirely of the cartilaginous vocal process of the arytenoid, really plays no part in voice production. The cords are simply brought into approximation and the membranous portion from the tip of the vocal process to the anterior commissure is the vibratory unit. Probably the localization of nodules at the junction of the anterior and middle third is a function of the fact that this is the point of maximum amplitude during phonation and therefore trauma is most likely to occur at this locus on the vocal cord. If one is strict in the use of the term "vocal nodule," limiting that diagnosis to true fibrous nodules, then it is apparent that voice rest alone cannot be sufficient management. Therefore, after a suitable trial of speech therapy has been attempted without complete resolution in patients who present with vocal nodules, surgery should not be delayed if restoration of a normal voice is to be achieved.

From the surgical standpoint, nodules are probably best managed by microsurgical technique, which allows very meticulous excision of the full thickness of the small knot of fibrous tissue with minimum trauma to the adjacent cord. It is important that the nonfibrous portion of the lesion adjacent to the nodule itself be removed also, either by microsurgical technique or with a laser. It

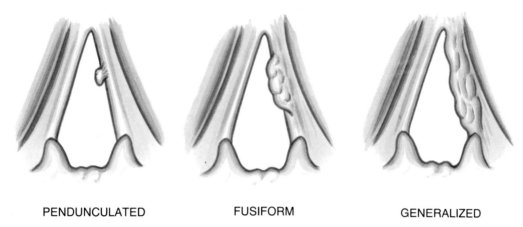

PENDUNCULATED   FUSIFORM   GENERALIZED

Fig. 3-22   Typical vocal cord polyps. Note the three most commonly encountered configurations.

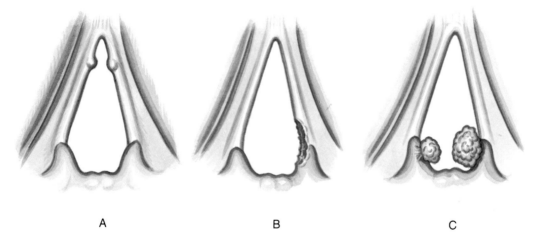

A   B   C

Fig. 3-23   (A) Vocal nodules. (B) Contact ulcer. (C) Granuloma.

has been my impression that the laser does not offer any significant advantages over standard endolaryngeal techniques in this lesion.

Contact Ulcer and Intubation Granuloma

Although these lesions are not identical, the pathophysiologic process from which they result is approximately the same. In both of these, the lesion is an area of granulation tissue resulting from trauma that has denuded the mucosa overlying a cartilaginous structure. In the case of contact ulcer (Fig. 3-23B), this is most commonly seen on the inner surface of the vocal process of the arytenoid. Granulomata, on the other hand, may be seen in this location, but are found on the inner surface of the bodies of the arytenoids (Figs. 3-23C and 3-25) as well. Contact ulcer occurs classically in the patient who is a high-tension, aggressive individual, or who uses a very loud voice for prolonged periods. The tips of the vocal processes become denuded because they are repeatedly driven forcefully together. Subsequent to the loss of mucosal integrity, the underlying perichondrial tissue becomes superficially infected. Because of the relatively poor blood supply to cartilage, the superficial infection prevents prompt remucosalization and thus favors the formation of a contact ulcer (Fig. 3-23B). Intubation granuloma, on the other hand, is usually the result of trauma to the arytenoids during endotracheal intubation. It may even occur in the absence of traumatic intubation. In particular, the use of assisted mechanical ventilation probably contributes to the formation of intubation granuloma because of the tendency for these flexible plastic tubes to slightly lengthen and shorten with increased and decreased intralumenal pressure. If the tube is not carefully fixed at the mouth so that it cannot slide in and out of the larynx even a millimeter or two during assisted ventilation, trauma to the posterior part of the larynx is likely to ensue, especially when one considers that most surgery is done in a supine position so that the tube tends to be forced towards the posterior part of the larynx. These lesions are likely to recur in spite of careful surgical and medical management.

The proper approach to them requires a combination of antibiotics, steroids, and, according to some authors, zinc sulfate, coupled with appropriate surgical excision if the lesions do not respond to medical management. Penicillin V, 250 mg four times a day for a period of 30 days, and steroids, such as Prednisone, 10 mg four times a day for a period of 10 days to 2 weeks, are a suitable medical regimen. This combination of drugs should serve to eradicate the infection and to reduce the excessive inflammatory response producing the granulation tissue. Whether zinc sulfate is actually helpful or not is open to controversy, which cannot be resolved here. I will simply report that zinc sulfate, 220 mg orally, three times a day, has yielded what appear to be dramatic results in a number of patients and, therefore, I use it routinely unless it is poorly tolerated by the patients.

If this medical regimen does not result in prompt improvement, it is necessary to resort to surgery. Although these lesions can be removed with microsurgical technique, it is technically difficult to get a good result, first because of the difficulty in

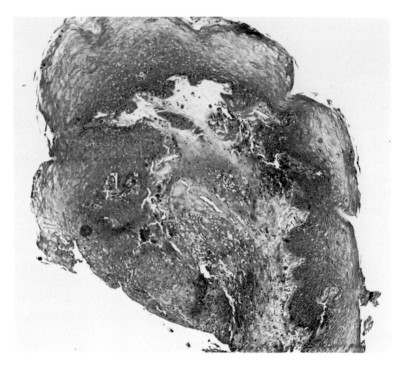

Fig. 3-24 Vocal nodule ("endstage" polyp). Note hyalinized dense fibrous tissue stroma.

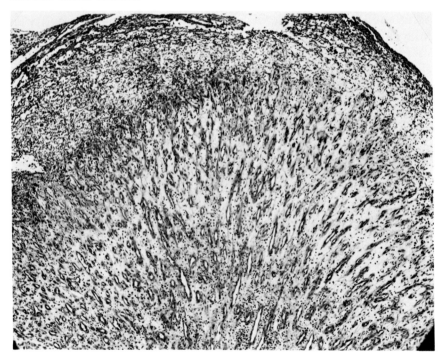

Fig. 3-25 Intubation granuloma. Note loose inflammatory stroma with multiple vascular spaces. The surface mucosa is either atrophic or missing altogether.

working in the posterior commissure with an endotracheal tube in place, and second because these inflamed areas in the larynx tend to bleed, making it difficult to be sure if all granulation tissue has been removed. For this reason, the laser has been a major improvement in the management of granulomata and contact ulcers. Not only does it permit the surgeon to remove every last vestige of granulation tissue with great precision, sparing the perichondrium wherever possible, but the laser has reduced bleeding to negligible levels, improving visualization. Probably most important, however, is the lack of damage to adjacent tissues so that healing can begin as promptly as possible. These lesions are a result of delayed healing and infection of the raw surface, so anything that will promote rapid healing will be advantageous. The laser does not provide an immediate cure in every case, but many previously intractable, recurring ulcers and granulomas can be managed successfully in this way.

Papillomata

The development of the CO_2 laser has revolutionized the management of this difficult lesion. If there is a single entity in which the laser is almost mandatory for adequate treatment, it is juvenile papillomatosis (Fig. 3-26 A and B). To begin with, the laser prevents most bleeding and therefore papilloma can be removed under direct vision with better preservation of normal laryngeal structures. Probably most important, however, is the fact that the laser destroys the involved cells with contained virus instantaneously with minimal trauma to adjacent cells and probably with minimal potential for spread of viral infection from involved tissues to adjacent uninvolved tissues. Thus, the laser can reduce the incidence of reinfection and therefore recurrence of the lesion, if indeed all affected tissue can be removed. Furthermore, because the laser is capable of removing large volumes of papilloma without producing significant edema in the residual tissues, tracheotomy can now be avoided in many more cases than was previously possible, thus avoiding infection and papilloma formation at the tracheotomy site and all of the other well-recognized complications of attempts to manage some of these patients by standard surgical techniques.

In severe cases where either a tracheotomy is still necessary or where one already exists, it is often possible to use the laser in retrograde fashion and remove papilloma from the under surface of the vocal cords from below as well as from above. The surgeon

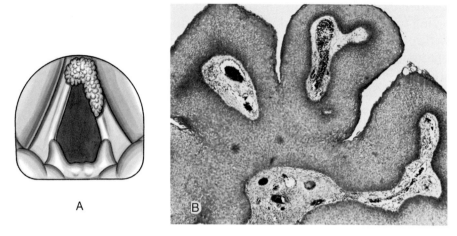

Fig. 3-26   (A and B) Laryngeal papillomata.

faced with massive involvement begins by removing as much as possible of what "doesn't look like normal larynx" and then waits a week or two for early healing to decide how much residual papilloma is present. It is more often the case that multiple applications will be needed to eradicate or control the disease then that a single one or two will be adequate.

In general, the aims of therapy in patients with juvenile laryngeal papillomatosis are as follows:

1. *Airway maintenance.* Exuberant growth of papillomata which occurs most often at the glottic level can result in decreased airway, especially in small children. The laser permits rapid removal of these lesions so that an adequate airway can be maintained with little or no bleeding and with so little edema that tracheotomy can now often be avoided where it would have been necessary before. When direct microsurgical technique is used, it is often considered wisest to remove only as much as is necessary to provide an airway, since it is almost impossible to be certain when normal laryngeal tissue is being injured in the effort to clean out all of the papillomata. With the laser, however, it is often possible to remove small bits of papilloma until everything is gone, leaving what appears to be a nearly normal glottic airway.

2. *Voice preservation.* Although these children suffer major interference with voice production, they will almost always develop normal speech patterns. It is, nevertheless, both psychologically and physiologically beneficial to try to maintain near normal voice production. Therefore, having once established

a satisfactory airway, the surgeon next must turn his attention to trying to restore as normal voice production as possible. To do this will require much more complete removal of papilloma than simple maintenance of the airway. In practice, most of these children are hoarse even after meticulous removal of papilloma, but the voice achieved can often be very satisfactory.

3. *Eradication of disease.* Needless to say, the surgeon would like to eradicate all papilloma so that they will not recur. This is sometimes possible, especially with the laser, but in practice even this instrument is not often curative after only one attempt. It is much more common to require repeated laserings or other means of removal from time to time. One may consider it a good result if the child requires endoscopic intervention only once or twice a year during the acute stages of the disease. There is strong evidence that juvenile laryngeal papillomatosis is of viral origin, but above and beyond this there is some suggestion that its ability to grow in certain individuals is related to immunologic competence. Many attempts have and are still being made to increase the ability of children so afflicted to diminish the growth of papillomata by improving their immunologic abilities. At the present time, none of these techniques is highly successful. Other approaches to papilloma management, including cryosurgery, ultrasound, autogenous vaccines, steroids, and so on, have all been recommended and have had claims of initial success made for them. A review of the literature, however, reveals that each of these techniques has fallen into relative disrepute with continued use. Now that the laser is available, they are of little or no value in the management of this disease.

In rare cases, despite aggressive management of the local lesion, there will be progressive growth of papilloma into the subglottic area and perhaps even down into the tracheobronchial tree. This will occur particularly when a tracheotomy becomes necessary despite other efforts, and the growth will often begin at or around the traumatized trachea. I have successfully managed one such case[7] by transecting the trachea below the lowest extent of growth and bringing out the two ends as a double-barreled tracheotomy. It was possible, after the papilloma had been controlled with repeated laserings, to reanastomose the trachea at a later date without serious side effect (Fig. 3-27 A and B).

Juvenile papillomatosis sometimes disappears at about the time of puberty. Although there is certainly a tendency in this direction, the trend is far from universal, and papilloma often persists to some extent even well into adulthood. What really seems to happen is that as individuals get older and have the papillomata

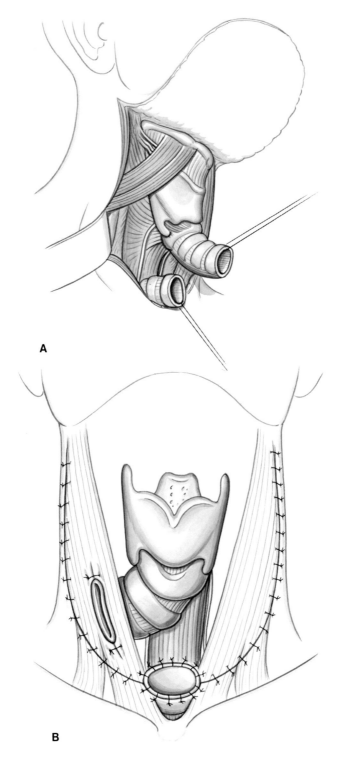

Fig. 3-27 (A and B) "Double-barrelled" (diversionary) tracheostomy. This technique may be useful in the management of exuberant papillomatosis as well as in cases of incompetent glottis.

for a long period of time, their immunologic response to this virus improves. Coupled with a larger larynx, this improvement permits more aggressive removal and eventually results in a static situation that can be considered a cure.

Premalignant and Early Malignant Lesions

The term *leukoplakia* should be restricted to clinical use and is intended to describe whitish plaques involving the mucosa of the larynx. Leukoplakia may be the result of hyperkeratosis with or without atypia, carcinoma in situ, early invasive carcinoma, or any of several other nonmalignant conditions that produce a whitish appearance (Fig. 3-28 A–E). A change in voice will be produced with any of these lesions, providing that the free surface of the vocal cord is involved. The diagnosis is made with indirect mirror laryngoscopy. In all cases in which an unexplained "white" lesion of the vocal cords is noted, complete removal by stripping will be necessary, both for diagnosis and management. Until the histologic nature of the lesion has been identified, it is unwise to observe such vocal cord changes even if they are known to have been present for many years.

Direct laryngoscopy can be performed by any of the techniques described earlier in this chapter and biopsies obtained accordingly. Since it is necessary to strip all the material from the larynx, the laser has proved extremely useful in the management of these lesions. The approach we now use is suspension microlaryngoscopy with meticulous stripping of all areas using microsurgical technique. When this has been completed, however, the entire raw surface of the larynx is carefully lasered to try to assure that every last shred of involved mucosa has been destroyed, leaving a healthy raw surface that can remucosalize, perhaps without recurrence of the lesion. The approach is the same regardless of the histologic diagnosis; that is, whether leukoplakia is due to hyperkeratosis with or without atypia, to carcinoma in situ, or even to microinvasive carcinoma. With the possible exception of this last diagnosis, most otolaryngologists would now agree that the proper management of this group of lesions includes meticulous stripping and observation to be sure that the regenerated mucosa is normal. If there is the slightest question that the healed mucous membrane harbors any persistent disease, repeat laryngoscopy and stripping is undertaken as often as is necessary. Stutsman[8] has shown that this approach to management yields a high cure rate with maximal preservation of a normal or near normal larynx, even in case of microinvasive carcinoma. The occasional case of premalignant or early malignant disease, managed in this way, that is desired to become invasive will be detected early in its course when it is still highly curable by either radiotherapy or appropriate surgery. Such an approach to management, however, mandates a reliable patient who clearly understands the need for meticulous and timely follow-up and the fact that repeated laryngoscopies and strippings may be necessary for some time. When, after suitable stripping, a normal or near normal voice has been achieved by this technique, the patient should be alerted to the fact that a change in voice may mean the lesion has recurred. Patients become rather sensitized to this and are often better watchdogs than the otolaryngologist.

Although the management of invasive squamous cell carcinoma of the vocal cord will be dealt with in more detail in a later chapter, a comment should be made about the use of the laser for endoscopic excision up to and including cordectomy. Strong[6] has now recommended that selected cases of invasive carcinoma of the vocal cord, T1 or early T2, may be managed by laser excision by an entirely endoscopic approach, thus obviating the need for hemilaryngectomy or radiotherapy for cure. Although early experience has been satisfactory and suggests that patients can be managed with as satisfactory a cure rate by this technique as by standard cordectomy, the voice achieved is usually not as satisfactory as would be expected after radiotherapy and even perhaps after cordectomy or hemilaryngectomy. Laser excision has several advantages to recommend it, however. The most important of these is the fact that it can be done entirely through the mouth, and often be done safely in patients who would otherwise not be a good surgical risk for open surgical procedures. In particular, elderly patients in whom the voice result is not critical should be considered for laser surgery rather than for radiotherapy for cure, since experience now suggests that older patients tolerate surgery generally better than radiotherapy.

Laryngeal Webs

It is possible to manage anterior laryngeal webs by entirely endoscopic means. This may be accomplished using a suspension laryngoscope and a Lewy arm. The larynx is exposed under general anesthesia, and the web is lysed either using microsurgical technique or with the laser. Following this, two 16-gauge needles are driven through the anterior neck skin in the midline so that the more inferior of the two passes just below the lower border of the thyroid cartilage, and the more superior passes through the

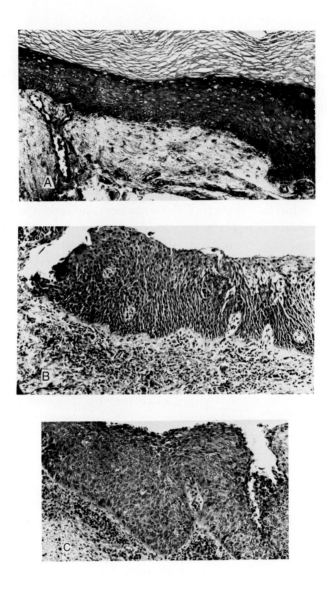

Fig. 3-28 (A) Hyperkeratosis without atypia. Note the thick keratin layer under which there is a normal sequence of maturation in the epithelium from the basement membrane to the surface. (B) Epithelial hyperplasia with atypia. Although the tissue is benign, there is not only thickening of the epithelium but a failure of orderly maturation from the basement membrane to the periphery. There is also some pyknosis and irregularity of the nuclei. (C) Carcinoma in situ. Although there is a clear malignant change in the mucosa, at no point is the basement membrane traversed. There is the usual inflammatory response adjacent to the rete pegs noted in one or two locations.

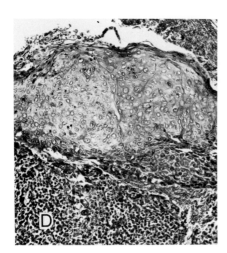 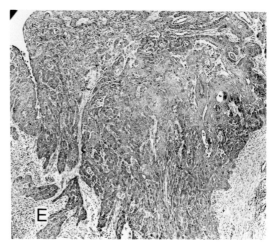

Fig. 3-28 (continued)   (D) Microinvasive carcinoma. This illustrates a picture very similar to carcinoma in situ. Note, however, the small nest of cells in the middle of the photograph invading beyond the basement membrane into the markedly inflammatory stroma. (E) Invasive squamous cell carcinoma.

thyroid notch precisely in the midline (Fig. 3-29). A fine wire suture is passed through each of these and grasped endoscopically by the surgeon. The wires are then led out through the mouth where each is fixed to a previously designed Teflon keel (Fig. 3-30). The keel is placed into the anterior commissure from above, while an assistant gently tightens the two wires to bring it into proper position and hold it there. The wires are then fixed to soft silastic buttons on the anterior neck skin (Fig. 3-31). The keel is left in place for approximately 2 weeks, following which it can be removed endoscopically. The idea behind this approach is to lyse the web and then to prevent reformation by interposing the keel between the two raw surfaces. Within 2 weeks, in most cases, one can expect remucosalization of the raw surfaces to a sufficient degree to prevent reformation of the web.

Advantages

The technique is entirely endoscopic and does not require any incisions in the neck skin. A tracheotomy is rarely necessary, providing a supramaximal dose of steroid is given intravenously 15 or 20 minutes before manipulation of the larynx is started.

Disadvantages

Although rarely reported, the possibility does exist that the wires might break and allow aspiration of the keel. An occasional patient will have sufficient interference with respiration that the keel cannot be tolerated without a tracheotomy. There is occasional infection of the deep tissues of the neck because of the conduit which the wire stay sutures provide from the laryngeal lumen out into the soft tissues.

OPEN SURGICAL TECHNIQUES

Obviously not all mass lesions that affect the voice can be approached endoscopically. Such lesions will usually be diagnosed by direct laryngoscopy and biopsy. Occasionally, even these will prove inadequate because of anatomic pecularities that make it virtually impossible to pass a rigid or even a flexible 'scope. In any event, all of the glottic larynx can be reached with good exposure via a transcervical approach. Since each of these techniques can be used for many lesions but generally are associated with a specific one, they will be dealt with accordingly.

Midline Thyrotomy

Small lesions of the glottic larynx, early carcinomas, and anterior and posterior laryngeal webs may all be approached very well via midline thyrotomy (Table 3-1). The technique is as fol-

TABLE 3-1   Surgical Approaches to
Various Laryngeal Lesions

Midline thyrotomy
   Glottic carcinoma
   Benign vocal cord lesions
   Anterior glottic web
   Lesions or webbing of posterior commissure

Lateral thyrotomy
   Laryngocele
   Tumors of false vocal cord

Transhyoid approach
   Posterior commissure
   Arytenoids
   Posterior pharyngeal wall

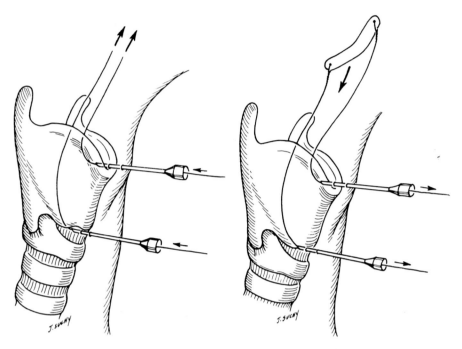

Fig. 3-29 Placement of 16-gauge needles above and below thyroid cartilage in the midline.

Fig. 3-30 Individually fashioned Teflon keel.

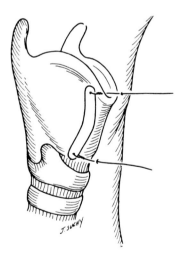

Fig. 3-31 Final positioning and placement of keel in anterior commissure.

lows: the neck is prepared and draped for sterile surgery, having first performed a tracheotomy. A midline incision is satisfactory, but not the most acceptable from a cosmetic standpoint. A modified apron flap incision is usually better, the two limbs being carried along the anterior borders of the sternocleidomastoid muscle and crossing the midline either at the level of the tracheotomy site or at the level of the cricoid cartilage. The flaps are raised in the usual subplatysmal plain to expose the strap muscles. These muscles are separated in the midline and retracted so that exposure from the body of the hyoid bone to the lower border of the cricoid cartilage is obtained. The perichondrium is incised in the midline and elevated for a short distance to each side. A cartilage cut is made precisely in the midline, using an oscillating saw (Fig. 3-32). The cricothyroid ligament is incised transversely at the midline for a distance of perhaps 4 or 5 mm to either side. A small microhemostat is placed through this incision from below, and the blades used to gently hold apart the undersurface of the vocal cords. Using a headlight, the operator now can look from below and see the undersurface of the cords, especially the attachment of the anterior commissure. A sharp knife blade is placed so that an incision can be made in the midline from below upward, through the midline cut in the thyroid cartilage. This is carried up to Broyle's ligament and continued directly through the midline to the base of the petiole of the epiglottis (Fig. 3-33). The incision can then be carried slightly to one side of the midline to reach the upper border of the thyroid cartilage. With this approach, it is possible to place small retractors into the larynx and to gently spread it so that the entire interior can be seen. Cordectomy for small carcinomas or less extensive resections for benign lesions, such as granular cell tumors, can be carried out via this approach. This technique can also be used to permit reconstruction of the larynx after trauma.

When the lesion for which midline thyrotomy has been performed is an *anterior glottic web*, the very act of opening the larynx in this fashion will, of course, lyse the web. Recurrence of the web can be prevented by placing a keel before closing the larynx. The author prefers to make the keel from a plate of soft tantalum cut at the time of surgery to appropriate size and provided with three small flanges. The keel is placed between the vocal cords, and the flanges are placed in contact with the cartilage beneath the closure of the perichondrium to hold it in place (Fig. 3-34). It is left in place for at least 2 weeks and is then removed under local anesthesia by incising the area directly. The

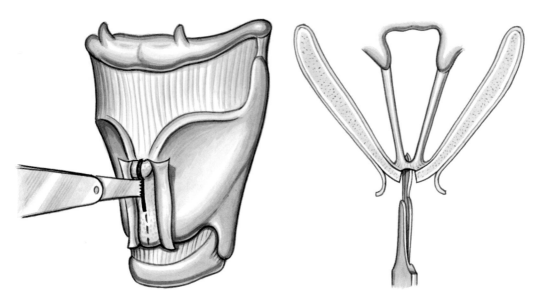

Fig. 3-32   Midline thyrotomy.

Fig. 3-33   Midline incision at anterior commissure.

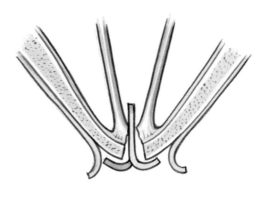

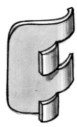

Fig. 3-34   Placement of midline tantalum keel.

keel is intended to permit remucosalization of the raw surfaces of the anterior portion of the vocal cords while preventing reformation of the web. It is advisable to place such a keel in all cases in which median thyrotomy is undertaken, except where cordectomy is performed. If this is not done, the incidence of blunting or webbing of the anterior commissure, resulting from the surgery, is significant.

Lateral Thyrotomy

The entire false cord, ventricle, true cord, and aryepiglottic fold can be approached through a lateral thyrotomy (Table 3-1). This approach is particularly useful and specifically designed for such lesions as an internal laryngocele and other tumors of the false vocal cord. It is possible to excise the entire lesion without ever entering the lumen of the larynx. This approach can also be used to visualize the opposite false cord, true cord, or arytenoid. The technique is as follows: a horizontal incision is made in a skin crease at the level of the upper border of the thyroid cartilage. Even though the lesion is unilateral, this should be a symmetrical incision that crosses the midline equally on both sides. The incision is carried through the skin, superficial fascia, and platysma, to expose the hyoid bone and strap muscles. The strap muscles can be separated in the midline and retracted from the side to be operated on, although they may also be transected and reconstructed at the end of the procedure. When the thyroid cartilage has been exposed and stabilized by placing double hooks behind it, an incision is made along the upper border of the thyroid cartilage from the base of the greater cornu to at least the midline on the involved side, completely through the perichondrium. The perichondrium is elevated from above downward to expose bare thyroid cartilage to approximately the level of the vocal cord (Fig. 3-35). Using the same technique, the perichondrium is elevated from the inner surface of the cartilage down to approximately the same level (Fig. 3-36). The exposed portion of thyroid cartilage may then be resected and either discarded or preserved for later use (Fig. 3-37). If the approach is being used for a lesion in the substance of the false cord (that is, an internal laryngocele or other tumor), it will be exposed in the process and can be removed by incising the inner perichondrium at an appropriate point and carefully dissecting out the lesion, staying outside the mucosa throughout (Fig. 3-38). In the case of an internal laryngocele, an effort should be made to identify the neck of the sac, which is usually located anteriorly at a point corresponding to the appendix

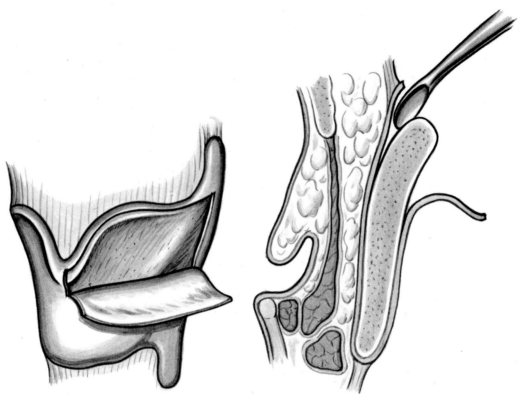

Fig. 3-35   Elevation of upper portion of thyroid perichondrium.

Fig. 3-36   Elevation of inner perichondrium to below the level of the true vocal cord.

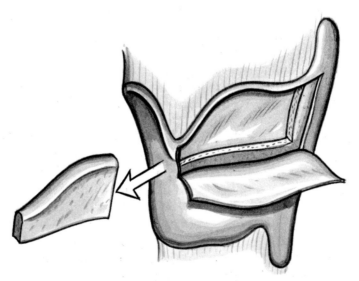

Fig. 3-37   Removal of portion of thyroid ala.

of the ventricle. A single pursestring suture can be placed to prevent leakage from within the larynx. In the case of minor salivary gland tumors, chondromas, and other benign or minor malignant lesions of the false cord, the lesion is simply excised. When this technique is used to expose the opposite side of the larynx, the surgeon incises the mucosa of the false cord and is then able to visualize the opposite true cord, the arytenoid, and the false cord (Fig. 3-39). The mucosa should be closed with fine absorbable sutures. Closure of the operative defect is accomplished by suturing the two leaflets of perichondrium to each other, using fine interrupted chromic catgut. A drain is placed in the neck, and the flaps and muscle are closed in the usual fashion.

Advantages

For lesions of the false cord or for internal laryngoceles, this approach has the distinct advantage of permitting excision without necessarily entering the mucosal-lined lumen of the larynx. When this can be done successfully, the possibility of infection is greatly diminished. Exposure is generally very good, and the procedure imparts little functional deficit.

Disadvantages

The internal branch of the superior laryngeal nerve is almost always injured or cut in this procedure, thus producing a sensory deficit on the same side of the larynx. In practice, however, this has rarely been a significant problem.

Transhyoid (Transthyrohyoid) Approach

The posterior portion of the larynx, particularly the interarytenoid area, can be approached satisfactorily and without risk to the anterior commissure via a transhyoid or transthyrohyoid approach (Table 3-1). In this technique a transverse incision is made at about the level of the upper border of the thyroid cartilage. The hyoid bone is exposed and an incision made down onto it to detach the infra- and suprahyoid muscles from the body of the bone. When this has been done the periosteum of the undersurface is carefully elevated and the mid portion of the hyoid bone is removed (Fig. 3-40). It is then possible to incise through its bed into the pharynx, which will expose the tip of the epiglottis (Fig. 3-41). The epiglottis can be grasped and retracted through the incision and by placing a retractor against the upper part of the incision the laryngeal introitus can be exposed. In lieu of this, one

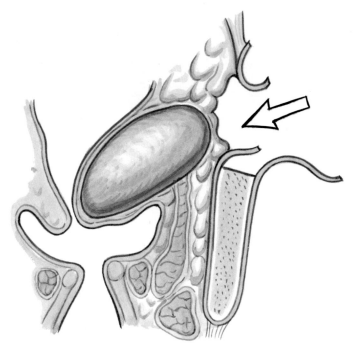

Fig. 3-38 Similar approach for excision of internal laryngocele.

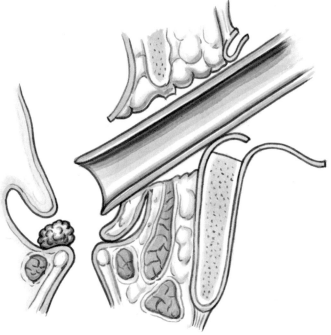

Fig. 3-39 Same approach for visualization of internal aspect of larynx.

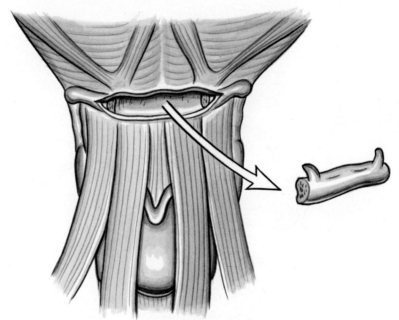

Fig. 3-40   Excision of midportion of hyoid bone.

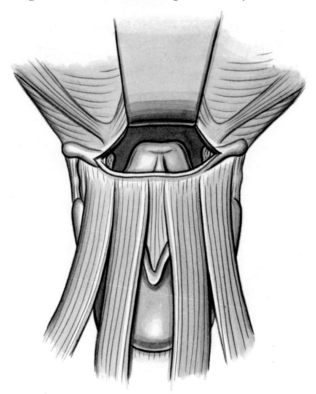

Fig. 3-41   Transhyoid approach to epiglottis.

can also simply incise the membrane between the hyoid bone and the upper border of the thyroid cartilage. However, this approach seems to provide less exposure than removal of the bone. Any surgical manipulations that are necessary can then be performed and the incision is closed by simply suturing the bed of the hyoid bone and repositioning the muscles into the defect, being sure to reattach the infrahyoid to the suprahyoid muscles directly. The bone itself need not be replaced.

Advantages

Avoids injury to the anterior commissure with possible subsequent webbing, gives excellent access to the posterior third of the vocal cords and the interarytenoid area.

Disadvantages

Limited exposure, poor access to the anterior portion of the larynx.

REFERENCES

1. Jackson, C. & Jackson, C.L.: Bronchoscopy, esophagoscopy and gastroscopy: a manual of peroral fundoscopy and laryngeal surgery, 3rd Ed. Philadelphia: W.B. Saunders Company, 1934.
2. Brunnett, R.E.: The pharmacology of drugs used in otolaryngology, Chap. 16. In English, G.E. (ed.): Otolaryngology, vol. 5. Hagerstown: Harper & Row, 1974.
3. Carden, E. & Crutchfield, W.: Anesthesia for microsurgery of the larynx. Can. Anaesth. Soc. J., 20:3, 378–389, 1973.
4. Jako, G.J.: Laser surgery of the vocal cords. Laryngoscope, 82:2204, 1972.
5. Strong, M.S., Jako, G.J., Vaughan, C.W. & Polanyi, T.G.: The use of the CO_2 laser in otolaryngology: progress report. Trans. Am. Acad. Ophthalmol. Otol., 82:595, 1976.
6. Strong, M.S.: Laser excision of carcinoma of the larynx. Laryngoscope, 85:1286, 1975.
7. Tucker, H.M.: Diversionary (double-barrelled) tracheotomy in the management of juvenile laryngeal papillomatosis. Ann. Otol., 89:504–507, 1980.
8. Stutsman, A.C. & McGavran, M.H.: Conservative management of superficially invasive epidermoid carcinoma of the true vocal cord. Ann. Otol. Rhinol. Laryngol., 80:507–512, 1971.

4 Voice Preservation in Management of Carcinoma of the Larynx

INTRODUCTION

Cure rates for new malignancies presenting primarily in the larynx have been improving steadily for the last three or four decades. This improvement has been due largely to better understanding of the nature of the disease, earlier detection, and better delineation of appropriate management for the different sites of involvement within the larynx.

Cancer of the larynx may be treated for cure in three basic ways (Table 4-1). The first of these is radiotherapy, the second is surgery, and the third is some combination of these two modalities, as a *planned* course of treatment. Each has its advantages and disadvantages, and one or the other may be more appropriate for an individual lesion, depending on the stage of advancement, the site of the lesion, and the age and general physical condition

TABLE 4-1   Treatment Modalities for Carcinoma of the Larynx

Radiotherapy for cure

Surgery ⟨ Laser / Conventional

Planned combined radiotherapy (pre- or postoperative) and surgery of the patient. With improving cure rates, attention has been turned to surgical methods that preserve all or at least some normal laryngeal function, in particular attempting to avoid the need for a permanent laryngostoma and total voice loss. Advances in this area have now reached the point where not more than one-third of all patients presenting with new malignancies of the intrinsic larynx should require total laryngectomy for cure.

Management of early glottic carcinomas has been discussed previously (Ch. 3, pages 46–47). The treatment of choice for T1 and some early T2 carcinomas of the glottic larynx is radiotherapy for cure (Table 4-2). If one averages the results reported for this

TABLE 4-2   Treatment Modalities for Carcinoma of the Glottis

T_1	Radiotherapy (vertical partial laryngectomy a good alternative)
T_2	Surgery (usually vertical partial laryngectomy)
T_3, T_4	High-dose *planned* radiotherapy and surgery (usually total laryngectomy)

modality in the current literature, an overall 5-year survival of roughly 80 percent can be achieved in this way. Of the 20 percent failures, approximately half can be salvaged by subtotal laryngectomy and most of the rest by a subsequent total laryngectomy, providing a determinate 5-year survival for all such patients that approximates 97 percent.[1-3] Most T3 and T4 lesions will be best managed by high-dose *planned* radiotherapy (either pre- or postoperative) in conjunction with total laryngectomy, with or without neck dissection. As such, these lesions will not be considered further in this text, since voice preservation is not possible after total laryngectomy. It can, of course, be *restored* after total laryngectomy in selected cases, surgical approaches for which will be considered in Chapter 5. If, on the other hand, subtotal laryngectomy is chosen as the initial treatment modality in T1 and T2 lesions of the glottic larynx, a determinate 5-year survival of approximately 90 percent will be achieved. Perhaps a third of the remaining 10 percent failures can still be salvaged by subsequent radiotherapy, and most of the rest by total laryngectomy. It follows, therefore, that the overall 5-year survival for T1 and early T2 lesions will be approximately the same, regardless of which initial modality is chosen for treatment. The real difference lies in the fact that if radiotherapy is chosen and is successful, the average resulting voice will be better than the average resulting voice after subtotal laryngectomy. On the other hand, a larger number of patients will ultimately require total laryngectomy for cure if radiotherapy rather than subtotal laryngectomy is chosen initially. Other considerations that must be taken into account include the patient's age, his general medical condition, and his social and economic situation.

Supraglottic carcinoma, on the other hand, carries a much more serious prognosis than most lesions of the glottic larynx. This is due largely to three factors: (1) the much richer lymphatic drainage of the supraglottic larynx; (2) the lack of early symptoms, in many cases leading to later detection; and (3) the less complete protective enclosure of the supraglottic larynx as compared to the cartilaginous "box" that encloses glottic carcinoma. As a result, these lesions tend to be more advanced when first seen, and with the possible exception of small lesions limited to the laryngeal surface of the epiglottis or occasionally of the false cord, radiotherapy alone rarely will yield 5-year cure rates equal to those for either surgery alone or combined therapy[4,5] (Table 4-3).

TABLE 4-3   Management of Supraglottic Carcinoma

T$_1$	Partial laryngectomy (conventional or laser) *or* radiotherapy
T$_2$-T$_3$	High-dose *planned* radiotherapy (5500r to primary and 4500r to both necks)
	and
	Supraglottic laryngectomy
T$_3$,T$_4$	High-dose planned radiotherapy *and* total laryngectomy
Neck dissection is also performed where indicated	

Neck node metastases will either be present when the patient is first seen or will occur at some time after definitive treatment in a relatively high percentage of supraglottic cancers. For this reason, the surgeon must be even more aggressive when considering the type of treatment to apply. Even when no clinically involved nodes are found, it will often be advisable to perform a *prophylactic* neck dissection or radiotherapy to the ipsilateral neck for all but the smallest primary lesions. Ample evidence now suggests that in the absence of palpable metastases, such prophylactic radiotherapy to the neck will obviate the need for radical neck dissection in most cases. When there are clinically evident neck metastases, high-dose preoperative or postoperative radiotherapy approximating 4500 rads to the neck and 5500 to 6500 rads to the primary lesion should be considered in conjunction with appropriate surgery.

Lesions limited to the supraglottic larynx, not involving the pyriform sinus or the base of the tongue, can be managed equally well by horizontal subtotal (supraglottic) as by total laryngectomy, provided certain factors of location of lesion are considered. Supraglottic laryngectomy is no different than total laryngectomy in the extent of tissue removed as far as the superior and lateral aspects of the resected specimen are concerned. It is only the inferior margin that must concern the surgeon in deciding whether or not a less than total procedure will suffice. Careful preoperative evaluation by laryngoscopy and, if necessary, x-ray studies should be carried out to be certain that at least 1- to 2-mm inferior margin will be achieved if the supraglottic structures are removed from the vocal cords at the level of the ventricle. In this regard, lesions of the false cord and aryepiglottic fold, and most of the epiglottis present no problem. Lesions that extend down along the petiole of the epiglottis are often difficult to assess, since they may extend into Broyle's ligament without this being suspected at preoperative evaluation. As a result, the surgeon should always have permission to perform a total laryngectomy even when it seems almost certain that a supraglottic laryngectomy will suffice. Whether or not preoperative radiotherapy has been employed, the technique for excision of the supraglottic larynx remains the same, although there may be some changes in reconstruction, depending on the lesion involved.

GLOTTIC CARCINOMA

When direct surgical intervention is chosen as the primary modality or, in selected cases, when an attempt at subtotal surgical salvage is assayed in the face of failed primary radiotherapy, several techniques are available to the surgeon. The decision as to the procedure most suited to the individual case will depend on how much, if any, preoperative radiotherapy was used, the general condition of the patient, and, most important, the extent of the lesion at the time that definitive resection will be undertaken.

Midline Thyrotomy and Cordectomy

For lesions of a superficial nature, limited entirely to one vocal cord with at least a 1-mm margin at the anterior commissure and which do not require excision of any more than the vocal process of the arytenoid, midline thyrotomy and cordectomy is an acceptable procedure. It is *contraindicated* in cases where motion of the involved cord is limited, due to either deep invasion of the muscle, or involvement of the inner perichondrium of the thyroid cartilage or of the cricoarytenoid joint. The procedure is relatively contraindicated in radiation failure cases since the denuded thyroid cartilage will be left in place and, in such situations, is subject to late radiation chondronecrosis.

Technique

A tracheotomy is performed in the usual location. Either a vertical midline incision or a small apron flap will give adequate exposure. The strap muscles are exposed and separated in the midline to give access to the thyroid cartilage. An incision is made in the anterior perichondrium of the thyroid cartilage at the midline and the perichondrium is elevated laterally for 1 or 2 mm in each direction (Fig. 4-1). Using a Stryker saw, the thyroid cartilage is incised in the midline from the thyroid notch to the inferior margin. An incision is then made transversely in the thyrohyoid membrane just at the midline. A small hemostat is placed through this incision and with a headlight, the operator looks from below upward to see the undersurface of the vocal cords. Using the spread hemostat to protect and separate the cords, a knife is inserted and the soft tissues in the midline of the larynx are incised from below, upward directly through the anterior commissure to the petiole of the epiglottis (Fig. 4-2). The separated halves of the thyroid ala may now be gently spread apart and held with small double hooks or retractors. This will give access under direct vision to the vocal cords on each side. The vocal cord and adjacent false cord can now be resected by elevating the inner perichondrium from the inner surface of the thyroid cartilage to separate all soft tissue from the cartilage (Fig. 4-3). The necessary volume of tissue is excised under direct vision, and bleeding is controlled with cautery. Ordinarily, no direct reconstruction is undertaken; that is, the raw surface thus produced is purposely left to granulate in and heal by second intention. Closure is accomplished by simply suturing the preserved edges of the anterior perichondrium to each other with fine absorbable sutures. The strap muscles are then reapproximated and the neck incision closed in the usual fashion with placement of a hemovac drain.

The postoperative course is usually quite benign, the patient being able to tolerate corking of the tracheotomy tube, usually in 3 to 5 days and removal of it at about 10 days after surgery. There is no real need to prevent oral intake of fluids and food beyond approximately 48 hours in these cases, since swallowing is rarely interfered with significantly.

Advantages

A fairly simple and direct procedure that can, if necessary, be done under local anesthesia, provides good exposure of the larynx and permits excision of small lesions under direct vision. Because the soft tissue is elevated in the subperichondrial plane, an assessment can be made at the time of surgery as to whether the thyroid cartilage is involved.

Disadvantages

The procedure should be undertaken with caution if more than a very superficial lesion is present, because involvement of the inner perichondrium is possible. In addition, it is probably contraindicated in radiation failure cases, since the remaining thyroid cartilage is likely to undergo chondronecrosis if previously irradiated. Probably the *major drawback* to this procedure is not that it is an inadequate cancer operation in properly selected cases, but that the voice results are generally less satisfactory than those achieved by standard hemilaryngectomy. This is probably due to the rigid lateral thyroid cartilage left in place, which prevents collapse of the lateral soft tissues and formation of a good band of scar tissue in the area in which the cord was excised. The absence of this "pseudocord" is probably the single most important factor in the relatively poor quality voice that results.

VERTICAL PARTIAL LARYNGECTOMY (HEMILARYNGECTOMY)

This procedure is *indicated* for primary or recurrent carcinomas of the glottic larynx, which can be excised by removing either the vocal process or, if necessary, all of the arytenoid posteriorly and which require excision of only a limited portion of the opposite cord. If achieving an adequate margin would require excision of roughly more than one-quarter of the anterior portion of the opposite true vocal cord, serious consideration should be given to near total laryngectomy with epiglottic reconstruction (as discussed in the next section). Extension of the lesion to a maximum of 1 cm below the free margin of the vocal cord is acceptable in unirradiated cases, but such extension should probably be limited to only 0.5 cm in cases that recur after radiotherapy.

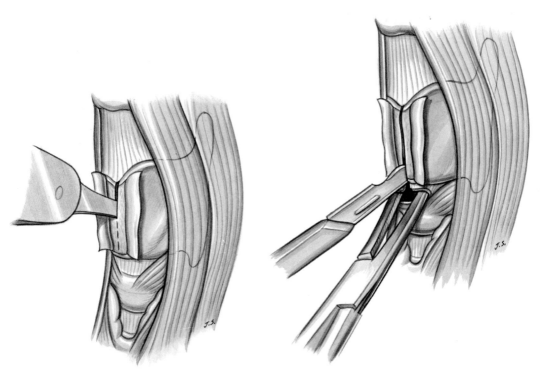

Fig. 4-1   Midline thyrotomy using an oscillating saw.

Fig. 4-2   A small hemostat is used to separate the halves of the larynx so that the midline can be incised with a knife from below upward.

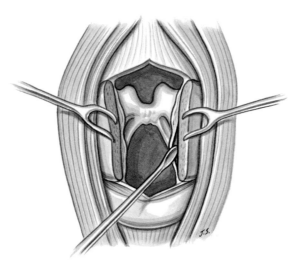

Fig. 4-3   Elevation of the inner perichondrium from the thyroid cartilage on the side of involvement.

When vertical partial laryngectomy is chosen, the technique that we prefer is as follows: a small apron flap is raised and a tracheotomy is performed in the usual fashion at the second tracheal ring. The larynx is exposed. The strap muscles are separated in the midline and retracted from the larynx on the involved side. An incision is made in the perichondrium at or slightly to the opposite side of the midline from the lesion and along the upper and lower borders of the thyroid cartilage (Fig. 4-4). The perichondrium is then carefully elevated back to approximately the base of the greater cornu to expose the cartilage itself. Using an oscillating saw, cuts are made first at the midline or slightly to one side and then posteriorly, just anterior to the base of the greater and lesser cornua, to leave a posterior strut to support these structures (Fig. 4-5). The cricothyroid ligament is then incised along the lower border of the thyroid cartilage, and through this incision the undersurface of the involved vocal cord is visualized by inserting a hemostat and spreading the soft tissues. The anterior commissure is then incised with a knife from inside out and from below upwards towards the undersurface of the cords, gently spreading the edges of the cartilage apart as this is done. The operator looks from below with a headlight until the edge of the cord and the lesion (Fig. 4-6) are seen. If the location of the lesion permits, the cut is continued right through the anterior commissure and Broyle's ligament to the petiole of the epiglottis, and from that point along the lateral margin of the epiglottis on the side of the lesion to the upper border of the thyroid cartilage. If the lesion extends to or slightly beyond the midline, the cut is moved appropriately away from it to allow at least 1 mm clearance. At this point, two halves of the larynx can be separated so that the involved vocal cord and the normal one to be preserved can be clearly visualized. With the scissors, cuts are then carried along the lower thyroid cartilage and upper border toward the posterior cartilage cuts (Fig. 4-7). If the lesion extends no farther than the tip of the vocal process, the vocal process is transected at its point of attachment to the arytenoid. If the vocal process or the body of the arytenoid are involved, then the arytenoid is disarticulated from the cricoid cartilage (Figs. 4-8A and B). The superior laryngeal artery is identified as it enters the larynx and is suture ligated. A posterior cut is then made, using an angulated scissors, from the lower incision to turn the corner into the posterior incision. The resection is completed by cutting along this aspect of the larynx to remove the entire specimen.

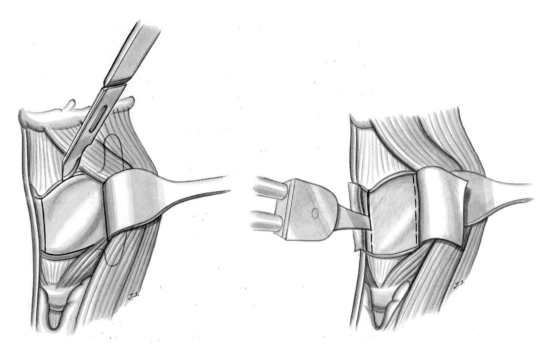

Fig. 4-4 Incision of perichondrium.

Fig. 4-5 Perichondrium reflected. Appropriate cuts are made in the thyroid cartilage with an oscillating saw.

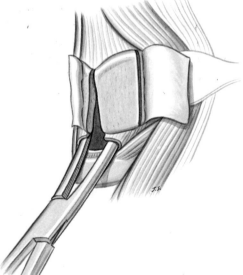

Fig. 4-6 Separation of laryngeal structures using a hemostat through the cricothyroid membrane. This permits midline incision under direct vision.

If the body of the arytenoid has been preserved, no reconstruction is really necessary. In fact, it is advisable not to try to remucosalize the raw surface thus produced, since this will interfere with formation of a pseudocord in this area. If the arytenoid has been removed, some bulk should be restored to the posterior part of the glottis to prevent possible aspiration. One useful technique is a pedicled muscle flap from the undersurface of the sternothyroid muscle.[6] An inferiorly based flap is elevated from the undersurface of the muscle, leaving it attached at the lower end (Fig. 4-9A). An incision is made into the preserved perichondrium in horizontal fashion at an appropriate point and the muscle flap led through it. The free end of the muscle is sutured to the remaining cricoarytenoid joint area and some mucosa from the pyriform on that same side is mobilized and brought forward to cover just the posterior part of the muscle (Fig. 4-9B). Following this maneuver, the perichondrium is closed, using interrupted sutures of 4-0 chromic catgut, from posterior to anterior and then along the anterior margin of resection, thus reconstructing the lateral laryngeal surface (Fig. 4-10). The strap muscles are then sutured loosely to each other. A small hemovac drain is placed and the skin flap returned and sutured in the usual fashion. No dressings are used nor are any antibiotics employed.

Most such patients tolerate the procedure extremely well with few, if any, complications. Swallowing is rarely a problem and the airway is almost always quite adequate approximately 7 to 10 days after the procedure. The patient is first extubated and, 2 or 3 days later, after the tracheotomy wound has been taped shut, the nasogastric tube is removed and the patient is fed.

Advantages

This technique provides the ability to adequately resect carcinoma of the glottis that can be encompassed with at least 1 mm margin within the limits described. Because the thyroid cartilage is removed, in effect providing a deep margin of resection that corresponds to the outer perichondrium, lesions with somewhat deeper invasion than could be managed by cordectomy, may still be resected safely in this way. The voice produced is generally superior to that to be expected from cordectomy, either by laser or surgical technique. There are few if any complications associated with this surgery in properly selected patients.

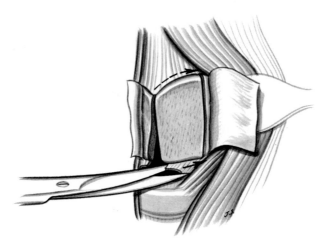

Fig. 4-7   Soft tissue cuts are made from medial to lateral using a scissors. This permits opening the larynx "like a book" so that the lesion can be excised under direct vision.

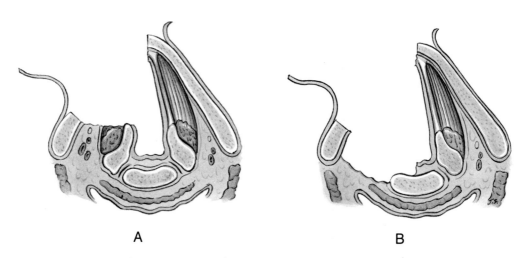

A   B

Fig. 4-8   (A) Defect produced when the arytenoid can be preserved. (B) Defect produced with disarticulation of the body of the arytenoid.

Disadvantages

The voice results are not as good as those generally expected after successful radiotherapy for cure.

NEAR TOTAL LARYNGECTOMY WITH EPIGLOTTIC RECONSTRUCTION

When a lesion of the glottis extends more than a millimeter or two onto the opposite vocal cord, near-total laryngectomy with epiglottic reconstruction should be considered if there are separate lesions on each cord or if one cord has frank, invasive carcinoma and the other carcinoma in situ or severe atypia.[7] Preparation of the patient and the surgical approach are exactly the same as for hemilaryngectomy.

The thyroid ala is exposed bilaterally by retracting the strap muscles. An incision is made in the midline through the perichondrium and along the upper and lower margins of the thyroid cartilage on each side (Fig. 4-11). The perichondrial leaflets are then elevated posteriorly on both sides to expose the entire thyroid ala. A cartilage cut is made on the side of greater involvement just anterior to the base of the greater and lesser cornua and on the side of lesser involvement at any appropriate point up to the same location (Fig. 4-12). The cricothyroid membrane is incised from the inferior margin of one cut to the other, and through this the undersurface of the cords is visualized. A scissors is used to transect the soft tissues medial to the cut on the lesser involved side, through the vocal process of the arytenoid, if necessary, or anterior to it if the situation permits, to reach the upper border of the thyroid cartilage. The cut is then carried along the superior edge of the thyroid cartilage on the lesser involved side, passing just anterior to the petiole of the epiglottis. When this has been accomplished, the thyroid cartilage can be displaced anteriorly and the opposite, more heavily involved cord, visualized through the defect. The incision is then carried along the upper border of the thyroid cartilage on the more involved side, until the cut on that side has been reached. Assuming that the margins are adequate, the excision of the lesion may be completed either just anterior to the body of the arytenoid, if the lesion permits, or, if necessary, by removing the entire arytenoid on the more involved side. The minimum tissue that must be left after this procedure should include the body of one arytenoid and a cartilage strut connecting the superior and inferior cornua of the

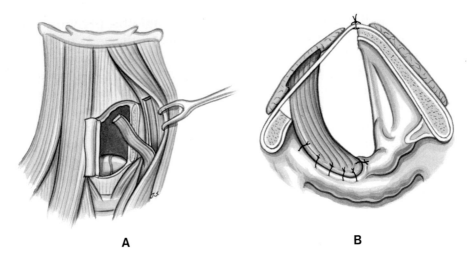

Fig. 4-9   (A) Inferiorly based muscle flap from undersurface of strap muscle. (B) Muscle flap sutured to bed of arytenoid cartilage.

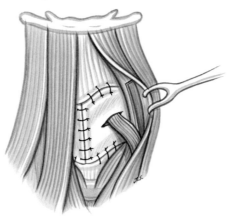

Fig. 4-10   Point of entry of muscle flap through perichondrium.

thyroid cartilage bilaterally (Fig. 4-13). The entire arytenoid, vocal process, and membranous on one side and all of the membranous cord and vocal process on the lesser involved side may be removed and satisfactory reconstruction still achieved. When bleeding has been controlled, the petiole of the epiglottis is identified and grasped with a tenaculum. The soft tissues of the pre-epiglottic space are separated with sharp and blunt dissection towards the reflection of the mucosa across the vallecula (Fig. 4-14). In the course of this dissection, the glossoepiglottic and hyoepiglottic ligaments will be encountered and may be cut. This maneuver will progressively mobilize the epiglottis, permitting it to be distracted inferiorly towards the cricoid cartilage. If a double hook is placed over the lower border of the cricoid to elevate it, and the epiglottis is pulled down with the tenaculum, the two can be made to meet. Using 3-0 or 4-0 nonabsorbable sutures, the free edge of the lateral margin of the epiglottis is sutured through and through to the cut edge of the thyroid cartilage remnants, *not* traversing the internal mucosa (Fig. 4-15). This closure is carried from above downward, and the lower margin of the epiglottis is then sutured directly to the remaining cricothyroid ligament, the stitches again being made to pass deep to the lining mucosa. With the surgical assistant relieving tension in the wound, these sutures are then tied one at a time from above downward. No attempt is made to close mucosa to mucosa. Rather, the redundancy of the excess internal mucosa will allow it to fall together, approximating the other side of the incision line and prompting good healing. The perichondrial leaflets that have been preserved are then brought to the midline over the epiglottis and sutured to each other to complete the closure (Fig. 4-16). The strap muscles are reapproximated, a small hemovac drain is placed, and the neck flap is closed in the usual fashion.

These patients are managed postoperatively exactly as one would a hemilaryngectomy patient. They rarely aspirate significantly and, if so, it is seldom a serious problem. The voice achieved in this procedure is understandably quite breathy, and there is rapid air escape. It is, however, in every instance distinctly superior to that to be expected by any patient with a total laryngectomy.

Advantages

All but a small portion of the glottis may be sacrificed and functional laryngeal reconstruction achieved. The procedure may be performed safely after radiation failure, or it can be used to salvage recurrences after previous subtotal laryngectomy.

Disadvantages

There is often some aspiration during early stages of swallowing, and the voice is rather weak and breathy.

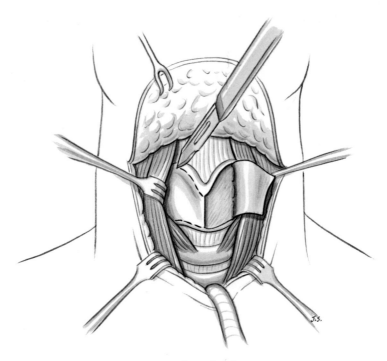

Fig. 4-11 Perichondrial incisions.

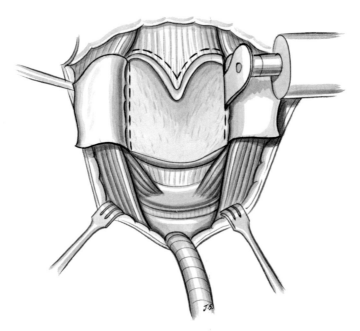

Fig. 4-12 Saw cuts using an oscillating saw.

SUPRAGLOTTIC LARYNGECTOMY

When lesions are limited to the false cords, aryepiglottic fold or epiglottis, *not* extending onto the base of the tongue, into the pyriform sinus or involving the body of the arytenoid, a horizontal subtotal laryngectomy (supraglottic laryngectomy) may be performed in properly selected cases. An apron flap incision is used. If a radical neck dissection is to be performed simultaneously, it may be an asymmetric flap wherein the limb on the side of the neck dissection is carried along the posterior aspect of the sternocleidomastoid muscle instead of the anterior border (Fig. 4-17). If this is done, it will rarely be necessary to employ an S-shaped extension in the supraclavicular area for exposure. The neck dissection is done first and left attached to the thyrohyoid membrane on the involved side. A tracheotomy may be performed at any time during the procedure that seems most appropriate to the surgeon.

The supraglottic laryngectomy is carried out as follows: the hyoid bone is grasped and, if the lesion is well away from it, preserved. If there is any question about involvement of the pre-epiglottic space or if the lesion comes close to the hyoid bone, it should be sacrificed. Using a cautery knife, the muscles are removed either from the lower border of the hyoid bone, or from the upper border if it is to be sacrificed. The greater cornu of the thyroid cartilage is exposed on the side of involvement, but usually not on the uninvolved side. This is done to protect the superior laryngeal artery, nerve, and vein in this area, which are so important to successful redevelopment of swallowing. The strap muscles are transected at approximately the upper border of the thyroid cartilage to expose it (Fig. 4-18). An incision is then carried through the perichondrium along the upper border of the thyroid cartilage, beginning at the base of the greater cornu on the less involved side, and carrying it across to the lateral aspect of the thyroid cartilage on the more involved side. It is also extended down the lateral border of the thyroid cartilage on the involved side, in the process detaching some of the inferior constrictor fibers from the cartilage (Fig. 4-19). The perichondrium is then carefully elevated from above downward to expose sufficient cartilage to allow the appropriate cuts to be made. The anterior commissure of the vocal cords will be found approximately at the junction of the upper and lower halves of the thyroid cartilage at the midline in males and at the junction of the upper and middle thirds in females (Fig. 4-20). When the cartilage has been ex-

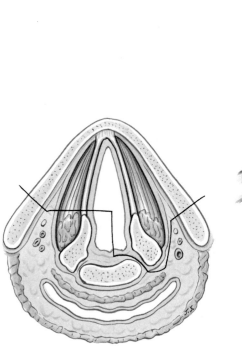

Fig. 4-13 Theoretical limits of excision. In selected cases an even more extensive procedure involving removal of the vocal process of the remaining arytenoid can be undertaken.

Fig. 4-14 Dissection of the pre-epiglottic space.

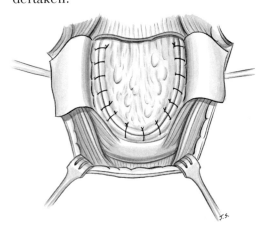

Fig. 4-15 Epiglottis sutured into place.

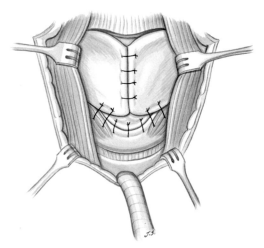

Fig. 4-16 Perichondrial closure completed.

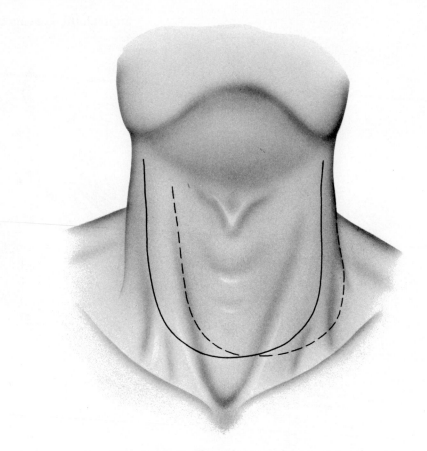

Fig. 4-17 Preferred apron-flap incisions.

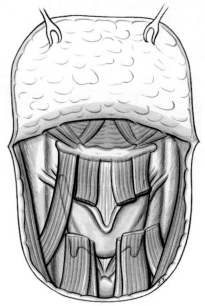

Fig. 4-18 Larynx exposed, strap muscles transected.

78

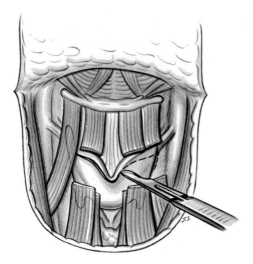

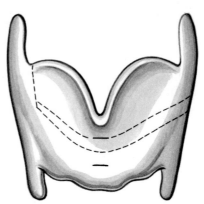

Fig. 4-19 Perichondrial incisions.

Fig. 4-20 Appropriate levels for cartilage cuts. The junction of the upper third and middle third of the vertical midline thyroid cartilage is used in females and in males in whom the thyroid cartilage is small.

posed, cuts are made from the base of the greater cornu, beginning at the upper border of the thyroid cartilage on the lesser involved side, and carried diagonally to the midline at the appropriate point. The cut continues transversely from this point to the base of the greater cornu on the lateral aspect to the thyroid cartilage on the involved side. With this skeletonization and mobilization of the structures to be removed, the surgeon may now decide where best to enter the larynx for exposure. If the lesion involves the laryngeal surface of the epiglottis or the false cords, it is best to enter through the vallecula. If the lesion is close to the vallecula, it is perhaps better to enter through the pyriform sinus on the involved side of the larynx, provided the lesion does not enter this area as well. Once an entry has been achieved, the opening is gradually enlarged under direct vision towards the known location of the tumor. This is done a bit at a time to allow the surgeon to gradually gain exposure of the lesion without approaching it too closely. When it has been exposed, the resection can be carried out to allow adequate margins. In most cases, supraglottic laryngectomy will comprise removal of the entire false cord along the anterior face of the arytenoid on the uninvolved side down to and through the ventricle on the uninvolved side, along the upper border of the true vocal cord to the anterior commissure, and from that point across the attachment of the petiole of the epiglottis, through the ventricle on the opposite side, to the face of the arytenoid. If the lesion is such that the arytenoid on the involved side does not have to be removed, the dissection is then carried along its anterior face to produce a mirror image of the dissection on the uninvolved side (Fig. 4-21). If the arytenoid must be removed, however, the vocal process is transected and the body of the arytenoid disarticulated in continuity with the specimen. The upper margin of dissection will be carried either just below or just above the hyoid bone, depending on whether this structure can be preserved. When the specimen has been removed and bleeding controlled, a cricopharyngeal myotomy should be performed. This is done by placing a finger into the esophageal introitus from above, palpating the cricopharyngeus muscle, and rotating the larynx with the thumb so that the posterior pharyngeal wall is brought into view (Fig. 4-22). A knife can then be used to carefully incise and transect all of the transverse fibers of the cricopharyngeus muscle so that nothing is left at that point but mucosa. If this is done properly, the creases of the operator's finger can be seen through his glove and the mucosa. Once the cricopharyngeal myotomy has been completed, the patient's anesthesia should be lightened to the point where movement of the endotracheal tube will produce movement of the vocal cords as the patient coughs. This is necessary to be certain that both cords are still innervated after the cricopharyngeal myotomy. If the recurrent nerve has been interfered with on one side, it is important to be aware of this at the time of surgery so that the paralyzed cord can be fixed in the midline to prevent later aspiration.

Closure of the supraglottic defect is then accomplished as follows: 2-0 or 3-0 black silk is used throughout. Sutures are placed between the remaining musculature of the base of the tongue (or if it has been preserved, the hyoid bone) and the free margin of the preserved perichondrium of the larynx below. The sutures are carried through the muscle of the base of the tongue at a distance of approximately 4 or 5 mm from the free margin, deep into the muscle but not through the mucosa and out through the raw surface of the muscle (or around the hyoid bone) without penetrating the mucosa (Fig. 4-23). Inferiorly, the stitch is carried through and through the free margin of the perichondrium. In this fashion, when the defect is closed the margin of the perichon-

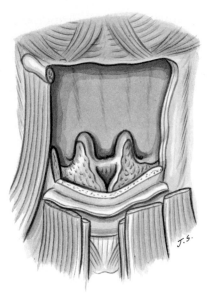

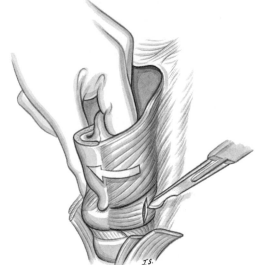

Fig. 4-21 Supraglottic laryngectomy completed.

Fig. 4-22 Cricopharyngeal myotomy.
Note rotation of laryngeal remnant to the
opposite side.

drium will be drawn up onto the raw surface of the cut edge of the
base of the tongue, pulling the overhanging mucosa down inside
the perichondrium for a short distance. In effect this creates a
situation analogous to the eaves of a roof. It is neither possible nor
advisable to try to bring the mucosa of the cut edge of the base of
the tongue down to the level of the true vocal cords. This will only
result in excess tension and a higher incidence of breakdown in
the wound. The stitches are placed from the side of lesser involvement to the side of greater involvement, being sure to approximate the midline of the base of the tongue to the midline of
the larynx. When two or three sutures remain as yet unplaced on
the side of greater involvement, a single corner gathering suture is
placed using heavier silk (Fig. 4-24). This stitch begins in the base
of the tongue, exactly as with the others, but is then carried as an
in-and-out stitch through the lateral pharyngeal cut until the free
edge of the perichondrium is reached, and then through it as well.
This will bunch and invert the tissue at the side of greater resection (Fig. 4-25). When this stitch has been placed, the remaining
two or three sutures left to be placed between the base of the
tongue and the perichondrium are put in. The stitches are then
tied one at a time, beginning at the side of lesser involvement.
The operating assistant crosses the next suture to take all tension

off the wound while each suture is being tied by the operator. When two or three sutures remain as yet untied on the side of greater involvement, the bunching suture and then the last two or three intervening sutures are tied. In this manner, if any stitch breaks during closure, it can be replaced. When the suture line is fully closed, the remaining strap muscles are approximated across it to take further tension off the mucosal closure. If the hyoid bone has been preserved, it can often be sutured almost directly to the remaining thyroid cartilage, thus reestablishing the relationship between the laryngotracheal complex and the base of the tongue, which can be very important to successful swallowing postoperatively. The neck incision is then closed in the usual fashion, covering the carotid with a dermal graft if a radical neck dissection has been performed. If preoperative irradiation has been employed and no complications have ensued, extubation may begin at approximately 2 weeks from the day of surgery. If the patient has not had previous irradiation, extubation may begin at about the tenth day. The tracheotomy tube is reduced to an uncuffed No. 4 and is then corked. When the patient can tolerate this for at least 48 hours, the tracheotomy tube may be removed and the wound taped shut. The nasogastric tube is then removed approximately 24 hours before the physician attempts to feed the patient. The necessary steps in retraining for swallowing have been outlined amply in the literature.

In cases in which both arytenoids may be left intact and normally mobile, the voice results after fully healed supraglottic laryngectomy are close to normal. If radiotherapy has been part of the treatment, persistent edema may create a problem in terms of swallowing, respiration, and even in voice. In any event, the resulting voice is usually very acceptable. Speech therapy is usually unnecessary following such surgery because, at least from a voice standpoint, the larynx is essentially functioning normally.

Advantages

Supraglottic laryngectomy has been shown to be at least as satisfactory as total laryngectomy in terms of long-range survival for properly selected lesions limited to the supraglottic larynx. The only real difference, from a surgical standpoint, between horizontal subtotal and total laryngectomy is at the inferior margin, where the remainder of the resection is the same as total laryngectomy. Provided the lesion has been properly assessed and an adequate margin of 2 or 3 mm achieved at the level of the true cords, cure rates should be roughly equivalent to total laryngec-

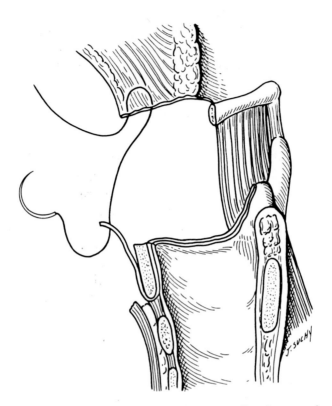

Fig. 4-23   Proper suture placement for closure of supraglottic laryngectomy.

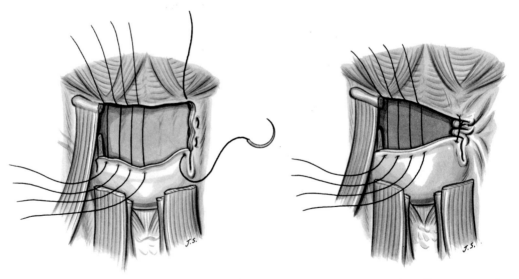

Fig. 4-24   Placement of "bunching" suture at lateral extremity of wound on side of greater involvement.

Fig. 4-25   "Bunching" suture tied.

tomy. Given such approximately equal cure rates, the voice that is preserved by performing supraglottic laryngectomy is clearly much superior to any restoration of voice by either pharyngeal speech or other surgical means that can be achieved after total laryngectomy.

Disadvantages

The patient who elects to undergo supraglottic laryngectomy must understand that there is an increased risk of delay in healing, fistula formation, and other complications of the surgery, plus the inevitable problem of learning to swallow properly again. Approximately 10 percent of all patients who undergo supraglottic laryngectomy never regain the ability to swallow sufficiently well to maintain nutrition and to protect the airway from aspiration. These patients may need to be subjected to a completion laryngectomy at varying periods of time after the initial surgery.

REFERENCES

1. Harwood, A.R., Hawkins, N.V., Keane, T., Cummings, B., Beale, F.A., Rider, W.D. & Bryce, D.P.: Radiotherapy of early glottic cancer. Laryngoscope, 90:465–470, 1980.

2. Ogura, J.H. & Thawley, S.E.: Surgery is the treatment of choice, Chap. 19. In Snow, J.B. (ed.): Controversy in Otolaryngology. Philadelphia: W.B. Saunders Co., 1980.

3. Espiritu, M.B. & Mathog, R.H.: Irradication is the treatment of choice, Chap. 19. In Snow, J.B. (ed.): Controversy in Otolaryngology. Philadelphia: W.B. Saunders Co., 1980.

4. Bryce, D.P. & Hawkins, N.V.: Primary radiotherapy for supraglottic laryngeal cancer, Chap. 13. In Snow, J.B. (ed.): Controversy in Otolaryngology. Philadelphia: W.B. Saunders Co., 1980.

5. Strong, M.S.: The case for combined radiation therapy and surgery for supraglottic carcinoma, Chap. 13. In Snow, J.B. (ed.): Controversy in Otolaryngology. Philadelphia: W.B. Saunders Co., 1980.

6. Biller, H.F., Ogura, J.H. & Pratt, L.L.: Hemilaryngectomy for T_2 glottic cancers. Arch-Otol., 93:238, 1971.

7. Tucker, H.M., Wood, B.G., Levine, H. & Katz, R.: Glottic reconstruction after near-total laryngectomy. Laryngoscope, 89:609, 1979.

5 Voice Restoration After Total Laryngectomy

INTRODUCTION

Despite the advances in surgical and radiotherapeutic capabilities that permit successful management of carcinoma of the larynx without resorting to total laryngectomy, the larynx must still be removed in a significant number of patients at some point in their management. The most widely accepted means of phonatory restoration for such patients has been pharyngeal/esophageal speech. Increased awareness of the need for professional rehabilitation, beginning preferrably in the preoperative phase, has permitted 40–50% of patients to recover their ability to speak—at least to levels satisfactory for reasonable day-to-day communication—after total laryngectomy. Serious attention must be given to early consultation between the speech pathologist and the otolaryngologist who anticipates the possible need for total laryngectomy in patients with cancer of the larynx. The speech pathologist will be best able to serve the patient if he or she has the opportunity to assess vocal quality, pitch range, speech capability, presence or absence of accent or regional speech variation, and so forth, before surgical intervention. Postoperatively, the surgeon must take an active part in psychological support of the efforts of the patient and speech therapist to achieve satisfactory speech.

In spite of these efforts, it will be necessary to provide an alternative means of communication for a significant number of patients. Such modalities as the electrolarynx, oral-stomal bypass mechanisms, signing, and the use of a pad and paper can be resorted to, but these are all less satisfactory than the ability to phonate and communicate in a more normal fashion. Clearly, the psychological, social, and economic status of each patient must be considered. The occasional elderly female, for example, who perhaps lives alone or has very limited contact with people outside the immediate family circle, may require relatively little ability to communicate verbally (although acceptance of such noncommunication may contribute to a further increase in isolation from society brought on by age).

In an effort to restore the ability to communicate verbally following total laryngectomy in patients who have been unable for one reason or another to develop satisfactory pharyngeal/esophageal speech, several techniques designed to recreate a connection between the respiratory system and the oropharyngeal cavity have been developed to permit sound production. Such techniques as those described by Asai,[1] Montgomery,[2] and others have in common the construction of a tubular connection, usually lined by mucosa or skin, between the laryngostoma and the hypopharynx. In theory, and to some extent in practice, all of these techniques work well if they are successful. Most of them, however, have suffered from the need for several stages, difficulty in keeping the constructed fistula open permanently, and/or aspiration through the fistula. Generally, these procedures are not well tolerated by patients who have undergone or will undergo radiotherapy as part of their management, and have not gained wide acceptance.

More recently, efforts have been made to develop a "pseudoglottis"[3-5] and, in a somewhat different approach, to construct a pharyngotracheal fistula that is used with a plastic prosthesis and thus does not suffer from closure or aspiration.[6] These two more recent techniques will be discussed in detail.

GENERAL CONSIDERATIONS

Even the most successful pharyngeal/esophageal speakers find it difficult to sustain speech beyond two or three words.

They must stop frequently to inject more air into the hypopharynx so that it can be expelled under controlled conditions and thus produce the necessary vibratory phenomenon in the active segment of the hypopharyngeal wall. Once this vibration has been successfully created, the resultant sound can be articulated and modified by the upper tract, tongue, lips, and teeth into intelligible speech. Pitch range is usually very limited and volume control is often a problem as well. The major difficulty, however, still revolves around the limited reservoir of air that can be achieved by injection into the upper esophagus and hypopharynx. Clearly, if connection could be safely reestablished between the respiratory tract and the hypopharyngeal vibratory area, improved restoration of speech would be possible. The general characteristics of a theoretically ideal restorative procedure after total laryngectomy is contained in Table 5-1. At the present time, no technique exists

TABLE 5-1   Criteria for Ideal Restoration of Voice After Total Laryngectomy

1. Single stage procedure
2. No aspiration
3. No prosthesis
4. No need to occlude stoma
5. Prompt return to voice
6. Sustained speech capability

that satisfies all of these criteria. Theoretically, laryngeal transplantation would satisfy these requirements in excellent fashion, but until the present this procedure has not been accomplished in humans and retains several, perhaps insurmountable, difficulties that prevent its use.[7]

The difficulties inherent in attempts to construct a suitable fistula connection between the respiratory and alimentary tracts are illustrated by the complications reported for most of the procedures that attempt to do this.[5] These include difficulty keeping the fistula open or, conversely, intolerable aspiration during swallowing through an overly wide fistula.

PSEUDOGLOTTIS RECONSTRUCTION

Serafini[3,4] has described a technique for pseudoglottis reconstruction which requires modification of total laryngectomy for its completion. Because cure of the patient is the first requirement placed on the surgeon in cases of carcinoma of any kind, it is not acceptable to diminish the necessary surgery in order to permit suitable reconstruction. Staffieri,[4,5] on the other hand, has described a technique that, with suitable modifications, can be performed without significantly limiting the surgery ordinarily done in total laryngectomy. It is this technique that is gaining the most widespread support in the United States at this time,[5] and which will be described.

Indications

Most patients with carcinoma of the larynx requiring total laryngectomy, with or without concomitant neck dissection, are potential candidates for neoglottic reconstruction. The procedure is contraindicated in patients with postcricoid or arytenoid involvement and in whom subglottic extension would require resection of more than one or two tracheal rings for an adequate margin. The procedure is performed at the time of total laryngectomy and adds only 15–30 minutes to the normal operative time.

Technique

A standard wide-field total laryngectomy is performed. The larynx is mobilized from below by transecting the trachea below the first or second ring, entering the space between the trachea and the esophagus, and dissecting the postcricoid mucosa off the surface of the cricoid lamina (Fig. 5-1). In this manner, maximum postcricoid mucosa is preserved, as permitted by the extent of the carcinoma. Once this maneuver has been completed, the remainder of resection of the larynx is not necessarily modified in any way from the usual technique. If it can be done safely, the hyoid bone is preserved. The remaining trachea is mobilized in the space between the esophagus and the posterior tracheal wall to permit formation of a permanent tracheostomy at the level of the third and fourth tracheal rings. This will be anchored directly to the skin, either through a matching excision of overlying neck skin or, in the case where an apron flap has been used, by placing the stoma in the incision line. At this point the preserved posterior cricoid mucosal flap is grasped and put on the stretch. A point in the midline of this mucosal flap, approximately corresponding to the center of the top of the transected trachea, is selected.

Using a cutting cautery, the muscle and submucosa is incised vertically (Fig. 5-2). The intact pharyngeal mucosa is grasped, pulled through the incision, and incised with the cutting cautery

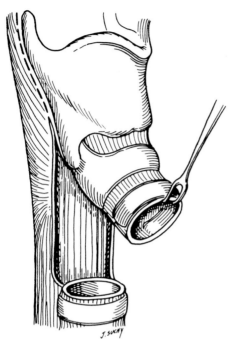

Fig. 5-1 Total laryngectomy from below upward. Note the party wall between the posterior aspect of the trachea and esophagus is maintained.

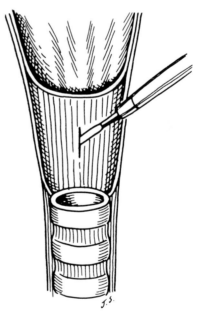

Fig. 5-2 Muscle and submucosa of the retained pharyngeal wall is incised vertically in the midline with the cutting cautery.

for a distance of approximately 8 mm (Fig. 5-3). The mucosa edges are then sewn to the submucosal and muscle layers with 4-0 silk. One suture is placed at each corner, at approximately a 45-degree angle from the longitudinal axis of the midline incision (Fig. 5-4). This is important so that the pull of the sutures will tend to draw the mucosal edges *together* rather than apart. The pharyngeal flap is then brought down onto the surface of the open end of the trachea and is sewn into position in two layers, using absorbable chromic sutures (Fig. 5-5). The pharyngeal defect is then closed in the usual fashion, as per the ordinary technique for total laryngectomy. If the hyoid bone has been preserved, it can be used as an anchoring point to attach the supraglottic musculature to the cut end of the trachea, thus reestablishing, to some degree, the normal relationship between the base of the tongue and the neoglottic reconstruction. When this can be accomplished, the base of the tongue will sometimes more effectively seal off the neoglottic opening during swallowing and thus minimize aspiration.

It is important that the patient be encouraged to relearn swallowing as early in the postoperative procedure as possible. The patient will have an easier time if the head is tilted forward during swallowing. In addition, it is helpful to teach the patient to take a deep breath and hold it during deglutition and then cough immediately after the swallow is completed to try to clear any of the material that may have collected on the neoglottic area. In this regard, the swallowing technique is no different from that used routinely after supraglottic laryngectomy.

Advantages

This technique, when successful, permits a one-stage rehabilitation of speaking ability without significant compromise of the standard total laryngectomy procedure for cancer. It adds very little time and no significant morbidity to the operation itself. The patient is able to produce sustained speech by placing his finger over the tracheostoma and expelling air through the pharyngeal fistula.

Disadvantages

Virtually all patients who undergo this procedure have some degree of aspiration. In many cases the aspiration is minimal and occurs primarily during eating. Therefore, it is manageable. On the other hand, it has required takedown of the fistula in some

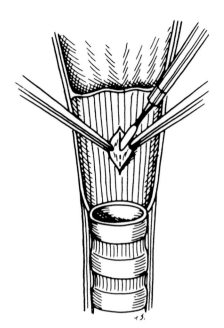

Fig. 5-3 Pharyngeal mucosa is pulled through the incision and then itself incised with the cutting cautery for approximately 8 mm.

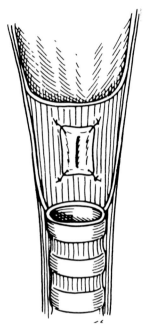

Fig. 5-4 Mucosal edges sutured to the pharyngeal musculature. Note that the stitches are placed at 45-degree angles to the midline so as to avoid distracting the edges of the wound from each other.

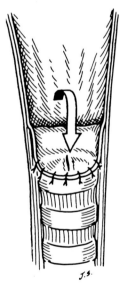

Fig. 5-5 Pharyngeal flap with neoglottic opening sutured to remaining anterior tracheal wall.

patients and has also been responsible for pulmonary complications in others. There has also been an increased incidence of poor primary wound healing with this technique, but it is difficult to determine if it is really statistically significant from the limited follow-up in the literature. Patients who have had preoperative radiotherapy or, to an even greater extent, who are planned for postoperative radiotherapy do not do very well. There is a tendency for the neoglottis to become edematous and even to heal shut while undergoing radiotherapy. In such patients, a string should be placed through the nostril, into the pharynx, through the fistula, and out through the tracheostoma so that it can be moved slightly each day to keep the fistula open until radiotherapy induced edema has subsided. Finally, because the operation should be done at the time of total laryngectomy, there is no opportunity to allow the patient to develop a good pharyngeal voice and thus avoid exposing him to the possible complications of the Staffieri neoglottic procedure.

THE "DUCK-BILL" NEOGLOTTIC PROCEDURE

Singer[6] has described a new modification of the secondary pharyngotracheal fistula procedure. Although at the time of this writing the procedure is quite new, we have had the opportunity to be trained in its performance by the originator, who has an experience of some 65 cases, and have now performed it ourselves in 15 cases. It is my opinion, at this juncture, that if this procedure continues to prove as successful in large numbers as it has in the first few cases, and carries with it the minimal complications observed thus far, it will become the procedure of choice for rehabilitation of speech in laryngectomy patients.

Indications

This technique is indicated in patients who have undergone total laryngectomy but have failed to develop satisfactory communicative skills by pharyngeal/esophageal voice or some other means within a minimum of 3 to 4 months of the time of surgery. Some authors prefer to wait 6 months to 1 year, to give the patient a better opportunity to develop pharyngeal voice and to rule out the possibility of recurrent malignancy.

Contraindications

This procedure is contraindicated if there is recurrent carcinoma in the area in which the fistula should be made or some other obstruction in the mouth or pharynx that would prevent speech development even if the procedure were successful. It is also contraindicated in patients who cannot safely withstand the minimal anesthetic and surgical intervention necessary. Females, as with the development of pharyngeal voice, do not generally do as well as males, but gender by itself is not a contraindication to the procedure.

The intimate involvement of a trained and knowledgeable speech pathologist is mandatory for the success of this procedure. Such an individual will be the primary factor in the acceptance and successful utilization of the prosthesis, once it has been placed.

SELECTION AND PREOPERATIVE PREPARATION OF PATIENTS

The patient is evaluated by an "air-blowing" test. The nasal fossa, oropharynx, and hypopharynx are anesthetized. A No. 16 plastic catheter is then placed through one of the nasal orifices and passed to a point in the pharynx below the level that corresponds to the mucocutaneous junction between the cervical skin and the tracheostoma. The catheter is progressively withdrawn while the examiner blows gently into it, thus inflating that portion of the esophageal/pharyngeal segment immediately above the opening of the catheter. The test is done to determine a "vibrating segment" within the hypopharynx, which will produce useful sound when inflated. The patient is usually asked to begin counting and to continue to do so while the catheter is slowly withdrawn to determine the most useful site. It is not uncommon, during such a diagnostic test, for the patient to go into pharyngeal spasm, thus making interpretation difficult. With experience, however, the examiner is usually able to separate these patients from those who have an anatomic stricture above the level at which the duck-bill prosthesis would be placed.

TECHNIQUE

Under general anesthesia, an esophagoscope is passed and the entire base of the tongue, oropharynx, neopharynx, and esophagus are examined carefully to make sure that there has not been unsuspected recurrence of carcinoma or a significant stricture. This esophagoscope is withdrawn and a specially adapted 9 × 11 mm × 30 cm adult cervical esophagoscope is introduced (Fig. 5-6). This esophagoscope has been modified by removing a "window" from its posterior surface near the distal end. Once the upper esophagus has been entered, the esophagoscope is rotated 180 degrees to bring the bevel posterior and the window anterior. The esophagoscope is manipulated to a point where the surgeon judges that the window lies somewhere posterior to the mucocutaneous junction of the posterior wall of the trachea. The exact site is determined by palpation through the tracheostoma. The assistant then holds the esophagoscope precisely in the midline. A 14-gauge intracath is bent into a gentle "C" shape (Fig. 5-7). A needle is then introduced through the posterior wall of the trachea approximately 3-4 mm below the mucocutaneous junction, exactly in the midline. The needle passes through the posterior wall of the trachea and the adjacent neoesophageal wall, enters the window in the specially modified esophagoscope, and is prevented from damaging the posterior wall of the esophagus by the esophagoscope. The intracath is then threaded through the needle proximally into the esophagoscope. It is grasped with a long esophageal forceps by the assistant and is led out through the mouth and clamped with a forceps. The needle and remainder of the intracath are cut off with a scissors, and the proximal end of the intracath, which is protruding through the laryngostoma, is also clamped. The end of the intracath protruding from the laryngostoma is then passed into the open end of a No. 14 plastic catheter. It is attached to the catheter by sewing it with silk sutures. A curved tonsillar forceps is then passed around the intracath through the puncture site to enlarge it, and the entire intracath with the following 14-gauge catheter is pulled through the mouth so as to introduce the larger plastic catheter through the puncture site up into the mouth, where it is held temporarily. An identical No. 14 plastic catheter is then passed through one nostril and grasped in the oral cavity and brought out through the mouth. The ends of the catheters are laid side by side and sutured to each other with 2-0 silk. The attachment is further assured by taping the two together with half-inch tape. The remaining free ends of the two catheters are likewise brought together in front of the patient, laid side by side, and sutured and taped to each other. In this fashion a circumferential loop is produced consisting of two No. 14 plastic catheters, one of which passes into the laryngos-

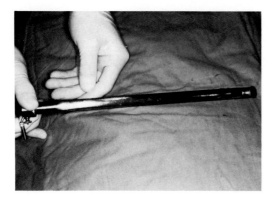

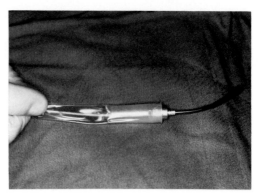

Fig. 5-6 Modified esophagoscope. This instrument facilitates passage of the modified intracath needle into the proper position. Please note, however, that an ordinary esophagoscope can be used by simply placing the Bevel anteriorly.

Fig. 5-7   Modified No. 14 intracath.

toma, through the puncture site, and up through the hypopharynx into the posterior oral cavity. Here it is attached to the second catheter, which continues out through the nasal cavity, and is finally attached to the other end of the first catheter (Fig. 5-8). The stent thus produced is left in place for 48–72 hours. The patient is kept NPO until the following morning when he or she is allowed to take food and liquids by mouth. To prevent crusting of the puncture site, cool mist is supplied via a tracheostomy collar, and the nurses are urged to give special attention to keeping the area clean.

Ordinarily the patient does not aspirate even liquids in the immediate postoperative period. If this should occur, however, the puncture site is cauterized with silver nitrate and the size of the plastic catheter is reduced to a No. 12. After 48–72 hours, the catheters are cut and withdrawn and a "dummy" duck-bill prosthesis is placed immediately so as to prevent aspiration and any contracture of the site.

Following this manipulation, the speech pathologist takes over and begins to determine the appropriate length of duck-bill prosthesis that will provide the best voice restoration for the patient. The prosthesis is placed under supervision and the patient is taught how to remove it and replace it for himself, as well as how to clean it. (Fig. 5-9 A & B).

Speech is produced by taking a deep breath and then occluding the tracheostoma with the thumb. Air is then expelled and forced through the duck-bill prosthesis into the hypopharynx at the appropriate point. This produces a good vibratory segment and with it a very satisfactory voice almost immediately. After a good voice has been produced (which may take from 3 to 7 days of practice), the patient is discharged with an extra prosthesis and the necessary cleaning equipment. In the beginning it is usually necessary to clean the prosthesis once or twice daily. The patient is followed on an outpatient basis at regular intervals until it is clear that he or she has mastered the care and utilization of the prosthesis. A period of 4 to 6 weeks usually is necessary before all postoperative crusting has ceased and the voice has stabilized. If the prosthesis comes out inadvertently, as will sometimes happen during coughing, or if the patient removes it and neglects to put it back, the puncture site will usually close within 2 to 4 days.

Advantages

This procedure is simple, inexpensive, and carries with it virtually no possibility of significant complication. It can be performed in patients who have undergone radiation therapy or for whom radiation therapy is planned postoperatively, although the incidence of prolonged crusting or swelling about the puncture site is increased during radiotherapy. The voice produced varies from fairly good to excellent but is superior to the best spontaneous pharyngeal/esophageal voice in almost all cases. Even when compared to the best esophageal speakers, the patient with a duck-bill prosthesis has a distinct advantage in that he can sustain speech for virtually as long as a normal individual and does not have to stop frequently for air injection. Volume control is usually quite satisfactory. Perhaps the greatest advantage of this procedure, particularly over other surgical means of voice restoration after total laryngectomy, is the fact that the curative surgery does not have to be modified in any way. Furthermore, since the procedure is done several months after the total laryngectomy, a decision as to whether or not the patient is likely to develop a good pharyngeal voice does not have to be made at the time of the original operation.

Disadvantages

The procedure requires a separate operation, although a small one, and also requires the continuous use of a prosthesis. Although the prosthesis is inexpensive and very simple, it has the

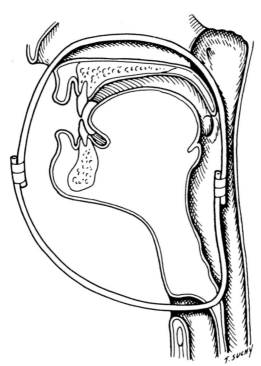

Fig. 5-8 Continuous loop of 14-gauge catheters in place.

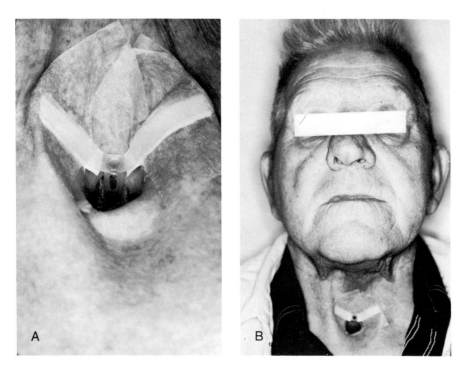

Fig. 5-9 (A and B) Duck-bill prosthesis in place.

potential to be lost, inadvertently expelled from the stoma, or even aspirated, although to the best of our knowledge this has not yet occurred. An occasional patient will have slight persistent leakage during the swallowing of liquids or saliva. This has been managed successfully in virtually every case by cauterizing or surgically diminishing the size of the puncture site and inserting a slightly smaller prosthesis. Finally, the patient must put a thumb or other occluding mechanism over the opening of the stoma, to speak.

Although there are many other means of restoring voice following total laryngectomy, I have selected the two presented here because they represent the most promising trends in current thinking on the subject. Neither of these procedures is totally satisfactory. Both have disadvantages, as has been pointed out. Nevertheless, by applying one or the other of these techniques, it should be possible to restore voice in almost every patient who has undergone total laryngectomy and has been unable to develop a satisfactory means of communicating without surgical intervention.

REFERENCES

1. Asai, R.: Asai's new voice production method: a substitution for human speech. Transactions of the 8th International Congress of Otology, Tokyo, 1965.
2. Montgomery, W.W.: Surgery of the Upper Respiratory System, vol. 2, Chap. 7, pp. 505–514. Philadelphia: Lea and Febiger, 1973.
3. Arslan, M. & Serafini, I.: Restoration of laryngeal function after total laryngectomy, report on first 25 cases. Laryngoscope, 82:1349, 1971.
4. Staffieri, M. & Serafini, I.: La Riabilitazione Chirurgica Della Voce E Della Respirazione Dopo-Laringectomia Totale. Association of Italian Otology Hospitals, 29th National Congress, 1976.
5. Sisson, G.A., Bytell, D.E., Beckes, S.P., McConnel, F.M.S. & Singer, M.I.: Total laryngectomy and reconstruction of a pseudoglottis: problems and complications. Laryngoscope, 88:693, 1978.
6. Singer, M. & Blom, E.: An endoscopic technique for restoration of voice after laryngectomy. Laryngoscope, 1980, To be published.
7. Tucker, H.M.: Laryngeal transplantation: current status, 1974. Laryngoscope, 85:787, 1975.

6 Preservation and Restoration of Voice After Laryngeal Paralysis

INTRODUCTION

In spite of ongoing efforts to alert surgeons to the risk of vocal cord paralysis, which may be encountered in such procedures as thyroidectomy, removal of parathyroid adenoma, anterior cervical fusion, and endarterectomy, there continues to be a significant incidence of surgically induced recurrent nerve paralysis.[1-4] Furthermore, increasing interpersonal trauma and high speed vehicular injury adds to the number of patients being seen with paralysis of one or both recurrent laryngeal nerves. Since the particular problems inherent in the management of patients with unilateral vocal cord paralysis differ materially from those of the patient with bilateral vocal cord paralysis, management of these two entities will be considered individually.

UNILATERAL VOCAL CORD PARALYSIS

The incidence of unilateral vocal cord paralysis as a result of thyroid surgery has been decreasing steadily.[1] At present, it would appear that the most common cause of unilateral vocal cord

TABLE 6-1   Unilateral Vocal Cord Paralysis: Etiology

	PARNEL AND BRANDENBURG (1970)	MAISEL AND OGURA (1974)	TITCHE (1976)	TUCKER (1979)
Thyroidectomy	17 (21%)	10 (8%)	5 (4%)	10 (5%)
Other trauma	2 (2%)	27 (21%)	18 (13%)	77 (37%)
Neurologic	3 (4%)	10 (8%)	21 (16%)	5 (2%)
Malignancy	32 (40%)	23 (18%)	51 (38%)	46 (22%)
Miscellaneous	27 (33%)	57 (45%)	39 (29%)	72 (34%)
Total	81 (100%)	127 (100%)	134 (100%)	210 (100%)

Tucker, H.M.: Vocal cord paralysis—1979: Etiology and management. Laryngoscope, 90:585–590, 1980.

paralysis remains idiopathic. Another almost equally common cause is neck trauma, including surgery other than thyroidectomy (Table 6-1).

Inadequate voice is the most common chief complaint of the patient who presents with a nonmoving vocal cord on one side. The voice is characterized by hoarseness, breathiness, and rapid air escape. Such patients will sometimes complain of being short of breath, but careful history taking will show that what they really mean is they must stop every few words to take a breath because they are unable to control rapid air escape. As a general rule, patients with otherwise uncomplicated unilateral vocal cord paralysis do not suffer sufficient airway restriction to be clinically significant. On rare occasions, particularly when the ipsilateral superior laryngeal nerve is also involved, the patient may complain of intermittent aspiration. This usually does not occur during swallowing but rather unexpectedly, due to aspiration of normal secretions, may occur at night while the patient is sleeping or in the middle of conversation. Most of these patients, however, will be seen because their voices are abnormal. Several factors must be considered in deciding which methods of management will be most appropriate for the individual patient.

When the cause of vocal cord paralysis is unknown, or is known but the recurrent nerve itself is definitely intact, no surgical intervention should be considered for a minimum of 6 months to 1 year from the onset of paralysis, unless serious aspiration occurs. In cases where the patient's livelihood depends on a normal or near-normal voice or occasionally for psychological reasons, early intervention may be justified, as considered below. It will generally be advisable, however, to put off any irreversible intervention until sufficient time has been allowed to elapse for spontaneous recovery and/or compensation. In a recent review[1] of over 200 cases of unilateral vocal cord paralysis, 64 percent were found to either recover or to compensate satisfactorily so that no therapeutic intervention other than speech therapy was needed. In fact, most cases of unilateral vocal cord paralysis can be improved, if not satisfactorily rehabilitated by speech therapy. It is important, therefore, that a speech pathologist be an early and integral part of the decision-making and management in every case.

When a sufficient period of time has been allowed to elapse and recovery or compensation has not been adequate enough to produce a satisfactory voice, three general approaches are available to the surgeon. These include: (1) Teflon (Gelfoam) injection, (2) surgical medialization of the vocal cord, and (3) reinnervation of the vocal cord.

Teflon (Gelfoam) Injection

Because of the peculiar anatomy of the cricoarytenoid joint (see Chapter 1), coupled with the residual adduction provided by the unopposed cricothyroideus muscle when the superior laryngeal nerve is intact, the unilaterally paralyzed vocal cord will come to rest in the paramedian position. As this is very close to the normal position for the vocal cord during phonation, the voice may not be very badly affected. Because of the flaccidity of the paralyzed cord, however, there is usually sufficient air escape and diplophonia that the resulting voice is noticeably poorer than that before injury. All means of rehabilitation, therefore, center around recreating the ability of the vocal cords to reach each other. Teflon injection must be considered the procedure of choice for voice restoration after otherwise uncomplicated unilateral vocal cord paralysis.

The procedure is performed as follows:[5] local anesthesia is desirable so that continuous voice assessment can be undertaken. This is important because Teflon is essentially not removable. Therefore, if an error is made, it should be on the side of conservatism. The patient is placed in the supine position and a standard anterior commissure laryngoscope is introduced. The paralyzed cord is visualized and the tip of the laryngoscope is turned slightly toward it so as to push back the false cord and fix the true cord in position by gentle pressure (Fig. 6-1). A Bruning syringe filled with Teflon is then introduced, and the needle is inserted into the substance of the vocal cord through its upper surface as far lateral as possible and between the tip of the vocal process in the lateral thyroid cartilage (Fig. 6-2). Teflon is then introduced into the proper position by squeezing the handle of the Bruning syringe until the surgeon feels that sufficient displacement of the cord towards the midline has taken place (Fig. 6-3). The instrument is then removed and the patient is allowed to phonate, taking care that the laryngoscope does not interfere with free motion of the mobile vocal cord. If necessary, an additional injection can be made at approximately the midpoint of the vocal cord, again as far laterally as possible in order to achieve a straight edge to the repositioned cord. Because edema will be produced almost immediately, the procedure should be carried out as quickly as possible, and the patient must be made aware that the voice achieved at the time of the Teflon is introduced may deteriorate slightly in a few days when the edema disappears.

Advantages

Teflon injection is inexpensive, performed under local anesthesia, and can be done without admitting the patient to the hospital. Moreover, the results, when successful, are almost immediate.

Disadvantages

Although proper Teflon injection will successfully medialize most vocal cords to the point where a satisfactory voice can be achieved, it does not restore the ability of the vocal cord to tense. The cord remains flaccid and may vibrate at a different modal frequency than the remaining innnervated cord. The slight diplophonia thus produced may be interpreted by the listener as roughness or hoarseness.

Teflon must be placed as deeply as possible in the muscle since if it is put near the surface, it may result in granuloma formation and extrusion of material. On occasion, especially if it is introduced into a partially functioning vocal cord, the material will be squeezed out of position and will need to be "touched up" from time to time in some patients. On rare occasions, Teflon has migrated into the subglottic area and has produced some airway restriction.

The advent of Gelfoam paste, which can be employed in a manner similar to Teflon, has extended the flexibility and usefulness of this technique.[6] Gelfoam, when injected into the vocal cord in an identical manner to that described above, will produce similar voice results. However, the Gelfoam will be gradually absorbed by the body and will have disappeared in from 6 weeks to approximately 3 months. As a result, it may be used safely in

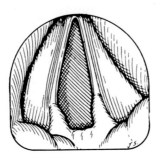

Fig. 6-1 Laryngoscopic view of paralyzed vocal cord. Note that the laryngoscope is rotated slightly to the side of paralysis to "fix" the paralyzed cord in position.

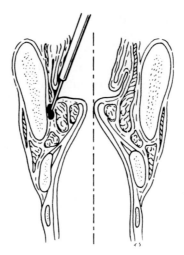

Fig. 6-2 Placement of Teflon or Gelfoam bolus. Note that the false cord is displaced as far laterally as possible and the bolus is placed as close as is possible to the thyroid cartilage.

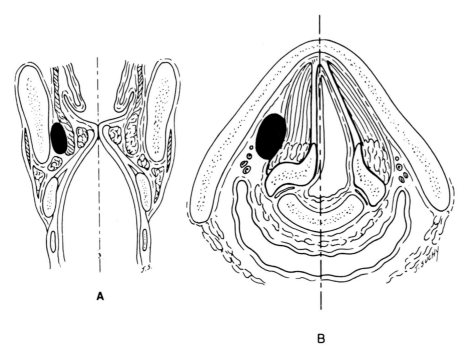

A

B

Fig. 6-3 (A and B) Proper placement of Teflon or Gelfoam bolus. Note that the bolus is placed as far posteriorly as possible so as to position it between the vocal process and the thyroid cartilage.

patients in whom prompt rehabilitation is desirable but whose possibility of spontaneous recovery still remains good. The patient who is aspirating or whose voice is absolutely necessary to his financial or emotional well-being can be considered for Gelfoam injection. The paste is prepared by using powdered Gelfoam. It is mixed with very small aliquots of sterile saline at the operating table until a quantity of semisolid Gelfoam, with a consistency similar to that of Teflon paste, is produced. It can then be loaded into an ordinary plastic syringe and from there inserted into the Bruning syringe. It is then injected into the vocal cord in exactly the same manner as described above for Teflon.

Surgical Medialization

In some patients with unilateral vocal cord paralysis, either because of simultaneous involvement of the superior laryngeal nerve or because of subsequent fixation of the cricoarytenoid joint, the vocal cord will come to rest at a point farther from the midline than is ordinarily seen with isolated recurrent nerve paralysis. In such cases the voice is even worse and aspiration may be a more frequent problem. It is the experience of many laryngologists that defects at the posterior commissure greater than 2-3 mm are difficult if not impossible to overcome with Teflon injection alone. For these patients, consideration can be given to surgical medialization of the vocal cord.

The technique we employ is as follows:[5] the neck is prepared and draped for sterile surgery. An incision is made in a skin crease on the side of paralysis, at approximately the level of the upper border of the thyroid cartilage, from the midline to a point just posterior to the anterior border of the sternocleidomastoid muscle (Fig. 6-4). Through this incision the strap muscles are exposed and retracted from the larynx. The upper border of the thyroid cartilage is identified, and a curved incision is made through the perichondrium of the upper margin of the thyroid cartilage from the midline to the base of the greater cornu (Fig. 6-5). The perichondrium is elevated from above downward to approximately the level of the thyroid notch. The inner perichondrium is likewise elevated from the inner surface of the same portion of the thyroid cartilage. The upper portion of the thyroid cartilage thus exposed is excised using either a scissors or a saw, depending on the degree of calcification (Fig. 6-6). The cartilage thus obtained is

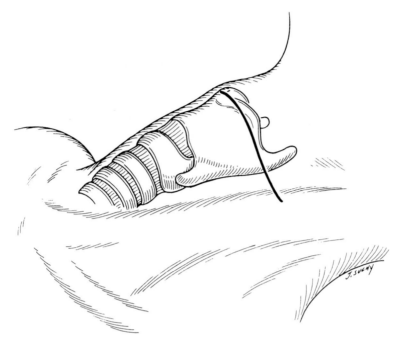

Fig. 6-4 Incision for surgical medialization.

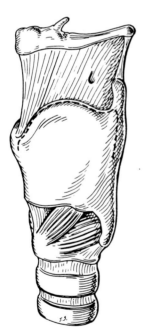

Fig. 6-5 Perichon-
drial cuts.

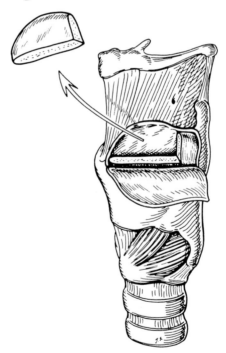

Fig. 6-6 Perichondrium elevated
on both sides of the thyroid cartilage to approximately the level of
the thyroid notch. The upper portion of the thyroid ala is removed.

105

modeled into a wedge for later reinsertion (Fig. 6-7). The perichondrium on the inner surface of the thyroid cartilage is carefully elevated down to a point below the level of the vocal cord, in the course of which a pocket is produced lateral to the vocal process and soft tissue of the vocal cord (Fig. 6-8). The wedge of thyroid cartilage is then inserted with the larger end posterior. This will effectively drive the vocal process and membranous portion of the vocal cord towards the midline (Fig. 6-9 A and B). The perichondrium is closed using interrupted sutures of absorbable 4-0 catgut and the neck is closed in the usual fashion after a small Penrose drain is placed. Tracheotomy is rarely necessary.

Advantages

This technique permits medialization of the vocal cord to the midline almost without regard to how large a glottic defect is present. It does not require insertion of any foreign material such as Teflon, although a subsequent small Teflon injection can be superimposed in those cases in which the voice results are still not completely satisfactory.

Disadvantages

It is sometimes difficult to be certain exactly how far to medialize the vocal cord, although observation through the laryngoscope can be helpful in this regard. It is occasionally necessary to add a small Teflon injection after the patient is fully healed to get the best possible voice results. This procedure, like Teflon injection, does not restore the ability of the vocal cord to tense. Hence, the resulting voice may still be diplophonic and somewhat rough, even when good strength has been restored.

VOCAL CORD REINNERVATION[5,7]

Patients with unilateral vocal cord paralysis in which the cricoarytenoid joint remains normally mobile may have restoration not only of the ability to bring the paralyzed cord to the midline but also to tense the vocal cord, if managed with unilateral vocal cord reinnervation. This procedure should be reserved for patients with particularly "valuable" voices, such as clergymen, actors, singers, lawyers, and so forth. The procedure is performed as follows: under general anesthesia the neck is prepared and draped for sterile surgery. With the patient paralyzed, and

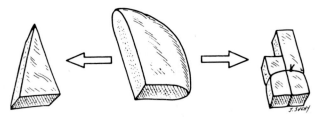

Fig. 6-7 Removed cartilage fashioned into a wedge.

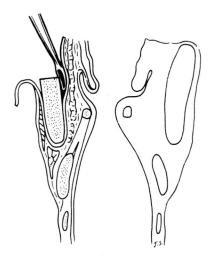

Fig. 6-8 Further perichondrial dissection towards the lower border of the thyroid ala on its inner surface.

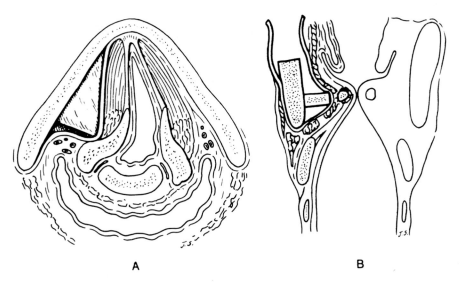

A

B

Fig. 6-9 Placement of cartilage wedge at the level of the true vocal cord.

before intubation has been undertaken, the larynx is exposed and the paralyzed arytenoid is palpated with a suction tip or other instrument to be certain that it is capable of being passively displaced to the midline; that is, that it has not become fixed as well as paralyzed. An incision is made at the level of the cricoid cartilage through a skin crease from the midline to a point just posterior to the anterior border of the sternocleidomastoid muscle (Fig. 6-10). This is carried through skin, superficial fascia, and platysma muscle to expose the anterior border of the sterno-cleidomastoid muscle. This muscle is mobilized and retracted posteriorly and the branch of the ansa hypoglossi to the anterior belly of the omohyoid muscle is identified as it lies beneath the fascia overlying the jugular vein (Fig. 6-11). If the nerve cannot be identified in this fashion, the omohyoid muscle itself is identified and its superior-anterior margin is mobilized, beginning as far medially as possible and progressing posteriorly until the nerve branch is encountered, usually with a small accompanying artery, as it enters the muscle on its undersurface. In either event, once the nerve has been identified and its action confirmed with a nerve stimulator, it is carefully mobilized back to its point of attachment to the main trunk of the ansa hypoglossi, which usually will provide adequate length for the procedure. A nerve-muscle pedicle is next designed, measuring approximately 2-3 mm on a side and encompassing the actual point of entry of the nerve into the muscle (Fig. 6-12 and 6-18). It is important that the muscle bundles be separated slightly because the nerve travels a short distance between the bundles before it begins to arborize (Fig. 6-13). If the proper point is not selected for the formation of the muscle pedicle, many of the necessary nerve fibers will not be preserved. When the pedicle has been produced and mobilized posteriorly, attention is turned to the larynx. The strap muscles are retracted and an incision is made through the perichondrium of the lower half of the thyroid ala. This is posteriorly based, begins approximately at the midline, and then is elevated posteriorly (Fig. 6-14). Using a Stryker saw, a window of cartilage is removed from the lower half of the thyroid ala, preserving an inferior and posterior strut (Fig. 6-15). The muscle that will thus be exposed immediately beneath the cartilage represents the most lateral fibers of the lateral thyroarytenoideus muscle, a major vocal cord adductor. The nerve-muscle pedicle is transposed into the defect and is sutured to the surface of the lateral thyroarytenoideus muscle using two 5-0 nylon sutures (Fig. 6-16). The perichondrial flap is then returned and sutured loosely in place (Fig. 6-17). The neck is closed in the usual fashion with a small Penrose drain.

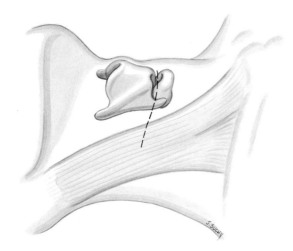

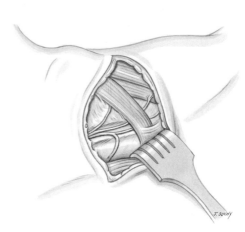

Fig. 6-10 Proper incision for vocal cord reinnervation.

Fig. 6-11 Exposure of the ansa hypoglossi and its branches beneath the fascia of the jugular vein.

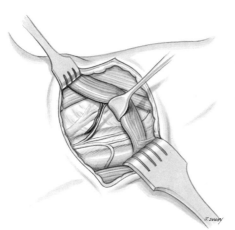

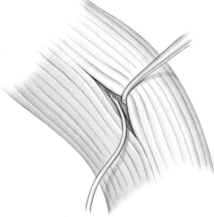

Fig. 6-12 Branch of the ansa hypoglossi to the anterior belly of the omohyoid. Note its accompanying small blood vessel.

Fig. 6-13 Exposure of nerve branch between muscle bundles. Note that the nerve travels for 2 or 3 mm between the muscle bundles before it begins to arborize.

Figs. 6-10 to 6-13 from Tucker, H.M.: Nerve-muscle pedicle reinnervation for vocal cord paralysis. Surgical Rounds: 14–21, July 1979.

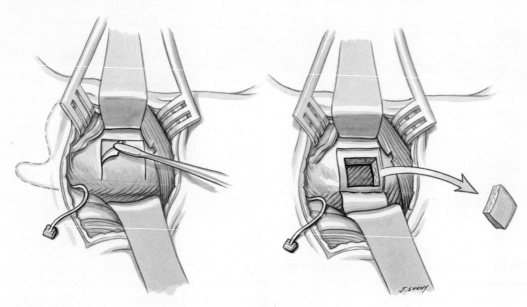

Fig. 6-14 Elevation of perichondrial flap.

Fig. 6-15 Removal of "window" of lower thyroid ala using an oscillating saw.

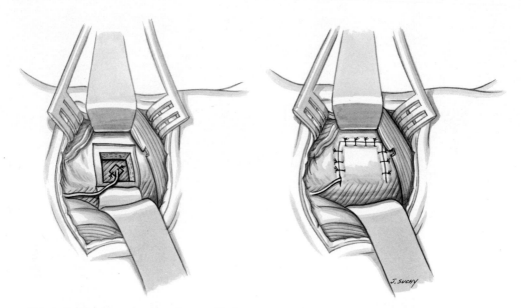

Fig. 6-16 Nerve-muscle pedicle sutured to lateral fibers of lateral thyroarytenoideus muscle.

Fig. 6-17 Perichondrial flap closed.

Figs. 6-14 to 6-17 from Tucker, H.M.: Nerve-muscle pedicle reinnervation for vocal cord paralysis. Surgical Rounds: 14–21, July 1979.

There will be some immediate improvement in voice in most patients mainly because part of the thyroarytenoideus muscle is detached from the thyroid cartilage, allowing it to medialize slightly. There may also be a certain amount of edema or fluid collection, which will also help the voice initially. The patient should be cautioned that this will be temporary and is not really the end result of the surgery. At a point in time varying from a minimum of 2 weeks to a maximum of 4 months from the time surgery is done, if it is successful, function will begin to return. This is manifested by any degree of motion of the reinnervated cord varying from rhythmic adduction during phonation to tonic adduction of the vocal cord to a more or less midline position. Even in this latter instance, EMG studies and direct observation have confirmed that the vocal cord is still able to tense during phonatory effort.

In a few cases, the degree of adduction that will be produced will still be insufficient for optimal voice results. In such a case consideration should be given to Teflon injection as an adjunctive procedure. Ten percent of the patients in whom this procedure has been performed have been complete failures; that is, there has been no visible return of function even 4 months after surgery. Speech therapy is mandatory in these cases, since the patient will require retraining in the ability to use the newly reinnervated vocal cord. Improved pitch control is usually the last thing achieved and may require several months after adductive function has returned.

Advantages

If successful, this is the only available procedure that not only restores approximation of the vocal cords but also the ability of the paralyzed cord to change tension during phonatory effort. As such, it offers improved potential for near normal voice restoration, although this is difficult to measure and document. Even if the procedure fails, either of the other two techniques mentioned above for voice restoration may still be undertaken. On the other hand, if Teflon injection or surgical medialization are undertaken first and are then unsuccessful, it may not be possible to subsequently reinnervate the vocal cord. Reinnervation can be undertaken even in cases where there is good potential for spontaneous recovery of function, since the recurrent nerve itself is not interfered with and no foreign material or cartilage has been placed into the substance of the vocal cord, which might interfere with good function.

Disadvantages

Reinnervation requires an open surgical operation and a wait of up to 4 months before any function returns. In at least 10 percent of all patients in whom it is undertaken, it will not be successful.

BILATERAL VOCAL CORD PARALYSIS

Inadequate airway is the primary presenting complaint of the patient who has bilateral vocal cord paralysis. In fact, the voice is usually fairly satisfactory because of the position in which the paralyzed cords fall because of the shape of the joint space and the unopposed adductive function of the intact cricothyroideus muscles. It is not uncommon for recovery room personnel to comment that they did not suspect a patient had bilateral cord paralysis (following a thyroidectomy, for example), because "his voice was good." Such patients often seem to have a reasonably adequate airway and only begin to manifest stridor and airway inadequacy when they either begin to have pain or try to exert themselves, thus putting more demand on respiratory capacity.

Patients with bilateral vocal cord paralysis may be managed in one of three general ways: tracheotomy, vocal cord lateralization procedures, and vocal cord reinnervation. Of these, only the first and the third address themselves to preservation of a normal or near normal voice. All of the techniques for vocal cord lateralization, including Woodman, Thornell, and laser excision techniques, are designed to do the same thing; to permanently abduct one of the paralyzed vocal cords to provide a satisfactory airway. As a general rule, the airway thus produced will be inversely proportional to the quality of the voice that results; that is, the better the airway the worse the voice. For that reason, whenever possible, methods of airway restoration that spare residual voice, or perhaps even allow for some degree of restoration, should be considered.

Tracheostomy is a part of the management of bilateral vocal cord paralysis in almost every patient. Even in patients who do not require tracheostomy for reasonable day-to-day respiratory function, it will usually be necessary to do one, if any means of surgical airway restoration is undertaken. Permanent tracheotomy should not be overlooked as a possible best means of management in carefully selected patients. Needless to say, it would be preferable for the patient not to have to go through the rest of life with an opening in the neck. Nevertheless, in elderly patients as well as in patients who are mentally retarded and in whom it is mandatory to preserve maximal voice capability, tracheotomy may be the most suitable means of providing a satisfactory airway. Indeed, if best possible voice is the patient's major concern, and if he or she is willing to have a permanent tracheotomy, it is even possible to consider Teflon injection or other means of surgical medialization of the paralyzed vocal cords, understanding that this will further decrease the airway, making the tracheotomy absolutely mandatory.

In most cases, however, when bilateral vocal cord paralysis has occurred, the airway will be less than adequate for reasonable day-to-day exertion. In such patients, existing voice can be preserved without further loss when nerve-muscle pedicle reinnervation can be performed.

The technique is as follows:[8] tracheotomy is performed if one is not already present. Under general anesthesia without intubation, the patient is paralyzed and the larynx is exposed with the laryngoscope. It is essential that both arytenoids be palpated carefully to determine that at least one, if not both, is passively mobile. It is interesting to note that approximately one-third of 200 patients with bilateral vocal cord paralysis seen by this author[1] had not only paralysis but actual fixation of the arytenoids, and this occurred in some cases as early as 6 months after the onset of paralysis. On the other hand, there were several patients with paralyses of 10–20 years whose arytenoids were normally mobile when palpated. It is advisable that the surgeon who is not experienced in this assessment should undertake to examine several otherwise normal patients who are being anesthetized for some other surgical procedure in order to get a feel for the ease with which normally mobile arytenoids can be displaced from the midline when the patient is paralyzed. If both arytenoids are fixed or severely limited in mobility and airway restoration is to be considered, the patient should then be left with a tracheotomy, or any of the several lateralization procedures mentioned above may be undertaken. If the arytenoids are mobile, however, reinnervation may be carried out at that time. The neck is prepared and draped on the side of better residual mobility for sterile surgery. A curvilinear incision is made in the neck at the level of the cricoid cartilage.[7,8] This is carried through the skin, superficial fascia, and platysma to expose the anterior border of the sternocleidomastoid muscle. In a manner exactly the same as that described for unilateral reinnervation, the sternocleidomastoid muscle is retracted and the branch of the ansa hypoglossi nerve to the anterior belly of the omohyoid is identified. The nerve-muscle pedicle, including the

actual point of entry of all of the major branches of the nerve into
the muscle, is produced measuring 2 or 3 mm on a side and put
aside as described above (Fig. 6-18). Using digital dissection, the
retropharyngeal space is entered and widely dissected so that the
larynx can be rotated as much as possible to expose its posterior
surface. This will be very easily accomplished in children and in
relatively young patients, particularly females. In older males,
where there has been extensive calcification of the ligaments and
other structures around the larynx, it may be quite difficult to
achieve. In any event, a double hook is placed over the lateral
border of the thyroid cartilage at a point just above the inferior
cornu. Using the thumb to push the larynx at its anterior commissure, the entire structure is then rotated so that the posterior surface is exposed to the operator (Fig. 6-19). With sharp and blunt
dissection, the fibers of the inferior constrictor muscle are separated at a point close to the inferior cornu and the reflection of
mucosa of the pyriform sinus is usually identified. This structure
is carefully mobilized and displaced superiorly (Fig. 6-20). The
muscle fibers immediately deep to the reflection of the pyriform
will be noted to be at right angles to those of the inferior constrictor. These are the fibers of the posterior cricoarytenoid muscle,
the only laryngeal abductor. If any doubt exists as to the identity of
this muscle, it can simply be traversed and the posterior wall of
the cricoid cartilage identified immediately below it. If the
operator now backs out one layer, he will have identified the
proper muscle. Since these muscles are not fasciated, no further
"roughening" or incision needs to be made. The nerve-muscle
pedicle is brought into position and is sutured to the surface of the
posterior cricoarytenoid muscle using one or two sutures of 5-0
nylon (Fig. 6-21). The larynx is then allowed to rotate back into
position and a small Penrose drain placed. The neck is closed in
the usual fashion. Postoperatively the tracheotomy is left in place
until it is satisfactorily determined that the patient's airway is safe
for day-to-day exertion with the tube corked for at least 72 hours.
Depending on whether or not the patient required a tracheotomy
before surgery, this will occur anywhere from 2 weeks to 4 months
after the surgery has been completed. If successful, function will
return somewhere in that period, and if it is not present by 4
months after surgery, the operation is considered a failure.

During this postoperative period, visible evidence of success
may be observed as follows: (1) approximately 40 percent of patients will demonstrate active abduction of the reinnervated cord
during one or more deep breathing efforts while sitting quietly in

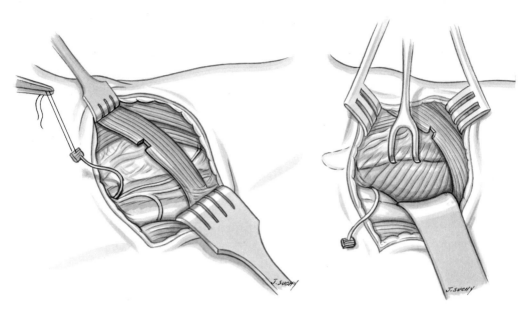

Fig. 6-18 Nerve-muscle pedicle produced from omohyoid muscle. Note that the pedicle measures only 2 or 3 mm on a side.

Fig. 6-19 Rotation of thyroid cartilage to opposite side exposing fibers of inferior constrictor muscle.

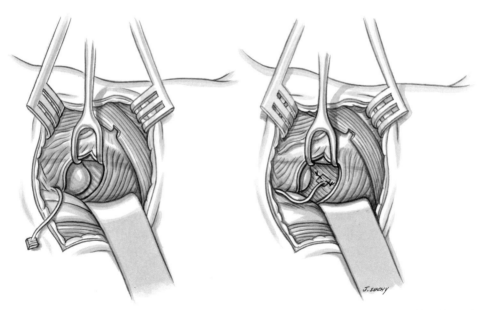

Fig. 6-20 Inferior constrictor fibers separated, exposing pyriform sinus.

Fig. 6-21 Pyriform sinus displaced superiorly to expose fibers of posterior cricoarytenoid muscle. Nerve-muscle pedicle sutured in place.

the examiner's chair; (2) most of the remaining successful cases will have motion in the vocal cord, either rhythmic abduction or tonic abduction, if they are stressed by vigorously running-in-place to the point where they pant heavily. The reason that some patients do not demonstrate abduction during quiet breathing is that the nerve-muscle pedicle is derived from an accessory muscle of respiration whose increasing activity is hypoxia dependent; that is, the greater the respiratory effort, the more active the nerve-muscle pedicle becomes. It follows, then, that if the patient has a glottic airway that is at least sufficient for quiet respiration, little or no motion may be observed under nonstressful circumstances. (3) In a very small percentage of patients, perhaps less than 5 percent, obvious clinical improvement becomes manifest by the patient's ability to exert himself satisfactorily without a tracheotomy tube when he could not do so before surgery. Yet, even with stress, it will be difficult to be certain that there is motion of the reinnervated cord. Previous observations both in animals and humans has demonstrated that in these patients, if the airway was totally occluded so that the patient was making maximal inspiratory effort against resistance, visible motion would be seen. This apparent lack of mobility may be explained on the same basis as (2) above; that is, the patient's degree of respiratory insufficiency is not enough to produce visible motion of the cord even when stressed. Nevertheless, such a patient would still be improved because he would have some additional ability under maximal need.

Advantages

When successful, this procedure restores the abductive capability of one or both vocal cords, particularly with increased demand. The procedure does not further compromise the voice remaining after bilateral vocal cord paralysis. Since the recurrent nerve itself is not interfered with nor is the passive mobility of the cord modified, this procedure may be undertaken even in patients in whom spontaneous recovery of one or both recurrent laryngeal nerves is possible. Reinnervation may be applied, for example, in the acute stage in patients who have sustained severe neck trauma, at the time a severed trachea is anastomosed, for example. Under such circumstances, it is inadvisable to explore the recurrent laryngeal nerves when preoperative paralysis has been noted, since either the nerves are severed, in which case they should not be reanastomosed, or the nerves are intact. Trying to identify them under traumatic conditions may result in further damage.

This technique has been successful in 90 percent of patients. More than 150 reinnervations have been performed by the author and the procedure has also been reported successful by others.[9,10]

Although it has not been undertaken as yet, it would be theoretically possible to further improve the voice of such a patient, providing the reinnervation achieved on one or both sides was truly excellent. This would allow the possibility that a Teflon injection or surgical medialization might be performed on the remaining paralyzed cord to better the voice, if the airway regained through reinnervation was deemed adequate. To date no patient in whom there has been successful reinnervation of one vocal cord has been willing to undertake the possible risks to try to strengthen the residual voice.

Disadvantages

The procedure has failed in approximately 10 percent of cases. Even in successful cases, a delay of up to 4 months may occur before function begins to return.

REFERENCES

1. Tucker, H.M.: Vocal cord paralysis—1979: etiology and management. Laryngoscope, 90:585–590, 1980.
2. Parnell, F.W. & Brandenburg, J.H.: Vocal cord paralysis; a review of 100 cases. Laryngoscope, 80:1036–1045, 1970.
3. Maisel, R.H. & Ogura, J.H.: Evaluation and treatment of vocal cord paralysis. Laryngoscope, 84:302–316, 1974.
4. Titche, L.L.: Causes of recurrent laryngeal nerve paralysis. Arch. Otol., 102:259–261, 1976.
5. Tucker, H.M.: Management of the patient with an incompetent larynx. Am. J. Otol., 1:47–56, Fall, 1979.
6. Schramm, V.L., May, M. & Lavorato, A.S.: Gelfoam paste injection for vocal cord paralysis: temporary rehabilitation of glottic competence. Laryngoscope, 88:1268, 1978.
7. Tucker, H.M.: Reinnervation of the unilaterally paralyzed larynx. Ann. Otol., 86:789, 1977.
8. Tucker, H.M.: Human laryngeal reinnervation: long-term experience with the nerve-muscle pedicle technique. Laryngoscope, 88:598–604, 1978.
9. Applebaum, E.L., Allen, G.W. & Sisson, G.A.: Human laryngeal reinnervation: the northwestern experience. Laryngoscope, 89:1784–1787, 1979.
10. May, M.: Rehabilitation of the crippled larynx. Laryngoscope, 90:1–18, 1980.

Index

Page numbers in *italics* designate figures; page numbers followed by t designate tables.